HIV/AIDS

Vulnerability in South Asia

HIV/AIDS
Vulnerability in South Asia

V. Ramamurthy

AUTHORSPRESS

Worldwide Circulation through Authorspress Global Network
First Published 2003
by Authorspress

E-35/103, Jawahar Park
Laxmi Nagar, Delhi-110 092

e-mail: authorspress@yahoo.com
quantum_soul@mantramail.com

Typeset in NewCenturySchlbk by Chitra Computers

HIV/AIDS: Vulnerability in South Asia
ISBN 81-7273-124-8

Printed in India at Tarun Offset, Delhi.

Preface

HIV/AIDS is one of the most dreaded disease of our century. The epidemic is unique in its devastating impact on the social, economic and demographic underpinnings of development. A decade ago, it was regarded primarily as a serious health crisis. Today, it is clear that AIDS is a development crisis, and in some parts of the world is rapidly becoming a security crisis too. There is now compelling evidences that the trend in HIV infection will have a profound impact on future rates of infant, child and maternal mortality, life expectancy and economic growth.

South Asia has 4.2 million people living with HIV/AIDS, equivalent to a prevalence rate below 1 per cent of the adult population. However, the relatively low prevalence disguises the presence of high risk factors which continues to make HIV/AIDS as significant challenge to development. HIV infection has taken root in South Asia, and poses a threat to development and poverty alleviation efforts in the region. The trend of increasing HIV infections, combined with heightened social and economic vulnerabilities that are fuelled by extensive commercial sex, injecting drug use, low condom use and access, and population movements highlights the need to act quickly and effectively.

What make people more fearful is that, after more than a decade of intensive research, medical science yet not find an ultimate curing medicine for the epidemic. However, experience has shown that prevention and intervention activities can successfully bring about reductions in HIV prevalence. The priority in the South Asian region is to implement HIV interventions among those sections of the population with high-risk behaviour, such as sex workers and their clients, injecting drug users, and migrant workers. There are, however, still many areas of concern. Interventions are needed urgently to prevent HIV-relating to injecting drug use and high risk sexual behaviour and to scale up the coverage of these interventions so that they have nationwide impact on the HIV prevalence.

Unless actions are now taken to scale up the response to curb the spread of HIV/AIDS, it could lead to significant economic and social consequences for all sectors. Because HIV/AIDS is not solely a health issue, an effective response requires a multi-sectoral partnership. Responding to HIV/AIDS now would cost only a fraction of what will be required at a later stage when the disease is allowed to become more widespread. International community as well as national governments have already took well-planned strategies and programmes, aiming to combat the pandemic from the face of earth. Within the framework of UNAIDS, World Health Organisation (WHO) plays a leading role in the health sector response to HIV/AIDS.

It is hoped that this book will contribute to a better understanding of the epidemic in the South Asia region and that governments, NGOs, policy-makers, anti-AIDS units and social workers will use the information it contains to guide them in better responding to the HIV/AIDS epidemic.

Editor

Contents

1

HIV/AIDS: Alarming Overview

HIV/AIDS is one of the most dreaded disease of our century. The epidemic is unique in its devastating impact on the social, economic and demographic underpinnings of development. A decade ago, it was regarded primarily as a serious health crisis. Today, it is clear that AIDS is a development crisis, and in some parts of the world is rapidly becoming a security crisis too. There is now compelling evidences that the trend in HIV infection will have a profound impact on future rates of infant, child and maternal mortality, life expectancy and economic growth. These unprecedented impacts at the macro-level are matched by the intense burden of suffering among individuals and households. Actions against the epidemic, in national as well international level have generated important insights into effective responses. While international political, financial and technical support are important, lowering incidence and mitigating the epidemic's impacts must be a nationally driven agenda. To be effective and credible, national responses require the persistent engagement of the highest levels of government.

PROCESS OF INFECTION

AIDS (Acquired Immuno-deficiency Syndrome) can take around 7-10 years to develop after infection with HIV (Human Immonodefciency Virus). HIV is transmitted through semen and vaginal fluids, infected blood and blood products, infected mother to her baby-before birth, during birth or through breast milk. A person who is HIV positive has HIV, the virus that causes AIDS. HIV damages the immune system, the part of the body that fights infection. Over time, the immune system becomes very weak. This stage of HIV is called AIDS. No one knows for sure when a person with HIV will get AIDS. HIV is different in different people. It can take a long time for HIV to make the person sick. Many people with HIV stay healthy for years. Understanding what it means to be HIV positive helps everyone. It helps people with HIV take the best care of themselves. It helps others give people with HIV the support they need and deserve.

Causes of Spread

AIDS spreads through:

i) Infected blood
ii) Infected needles
iii) Multiple partners
iv) Infected mother to her baby before birth
v) Injectable drug abuse

HIV can be passed on because the virus is present in the sexual fluids and blood of infected people. If infected blood or sexual fluid gets into your blood, then you will become infected. If a man with HIV has vaginal intercourse without a condom, infected fluid could pass into the woman's blood stream through a tiny cut or sore inside her body. This can be so small that you don't know about it. If a couple have anal intercourse the risk of infection is greater than with vaginal intercourse. If a woman with HIV has sexual intercourse without a condom, HIV could get into the man's blood through a sore patch on his penis or by getting into the tube which runs down the penis. If there is any contact with blood during sex, this increases the risk of infection. For example, there may be blood in the vagina if intercourse happens during a woman's period. There can also be bleeding during anal intercourse.

The AIDS virus causes a weakness of the immune system. When it infects the body, it prefers to attack certain cells of our defence system. These cells are called helper T cells which are a fundamental part of our immune system. The AIDS virus almost fully specialises on these white blood cells (WBC) since these helper T cells have CD4 molecules on the surface to which the AIDS virus binds.

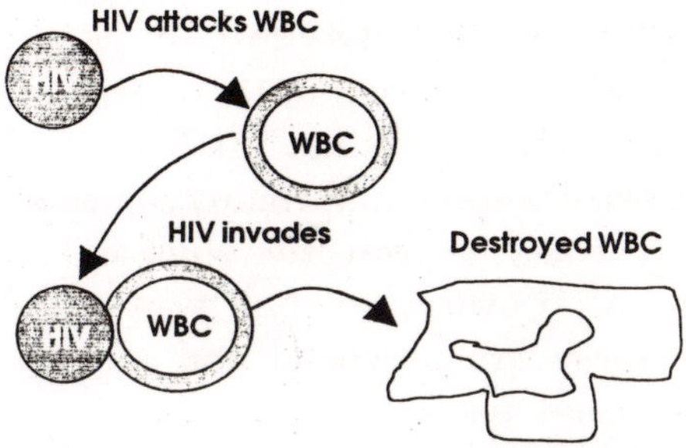

Figure 1: Dagrammatic representation of HIV's attack on WBC

The AIDS virus, to put it simply, consists of genetic information on the inside and a protective outer shell of proteins and glycoproteins. Since viruses use the host cell's resources for reproduction, they don't need to contribute much themselves. That's why they are much smaller than the host cells, e.g. helper T cells. In the host cell's nucleus, there are more than 100,000 times as much genetic information stored than under the protein shell of the AIDS virus. However, there is no way for the host cell to stop the virus once the cell has been infected.

The infection proceeds in this manner: The virus anchors itself to a special protein (CD4) on the surface of the helper T cell. This causes the viral membrane to fuse with the host cell's membrane. This way the genetic information gets inside the cell. The AIDS virus belongs to a special group of viruses. Its genetic information is not encoded as DNA, but instead as RNA (ribonucleic acid) and therefore has to be reverse transcripted into DNA. The tools for this are delivered by the host cell itself, except for a little helper protein (reverse transcriptase) which the virus has brought with itself. The DNA is now legible for the cell and is transferred to the nucleus. This process is already finished by a half of a day after infection. The foreign piece of DNA is then inserted randomly into the host DNA and it is now ready to be transcribed. At the beginning of AIDS, the viral DNA is being transcribed to form many RNA molecules—the signal which causes this is yet unknown.

The accruing RNA is carried to the cytoplasm of the cell, where it can start making proteins. The RNA, with the help of the host's resources, begins to make many copies of the different parts of the AIDS virus (the protective shell and the helper and anchor proteins). After everything has been copied, thousands of bubbles like these are produced and migrate to the cell membrane surface and fuse with it.

Finally, a copy of the RNA genetic information is added to the bubble. Then this section of the cell membrane turns inside out and new viruses leave the cell. Naturally, the release of the new AIDS viruses significantly weakens the host cell which soon dies. As a result the immune system weakens and AIDS starts. In early 1996 there were 28m people infected worldwide. This number includes people who already died of AIDS. These numbers do not include the number of people who already died.

SYMPTOMS OF AIDS

The general symptoms of AIDS are:

— prolonged, unexplained fatigue
— swollen glands (lymph nodes)
— fever lasting more than 10 days
— chills
— excessive sweating especially night sweats

— mouth lesions including yeast lesions and painful, swollen gums
— sore throat
— cough
— shortness of breath
— changes in bowel habits including constipation
— frequent diarrhoea
— symptoms of a specific opportunistic infection (such as candida, pneumocystis, and so on)
— tumour (*Kaposi* sarcoma)
— skin rashes or lesions of various types
— unintentional weight loss
— general discomfort or uneasiness (malaise)
— headache

Additional symptoms that may be associated with this disease:

— speech impairment
— muscle atrophy
— memory loss
— decreasing intellectual function
— joint swelling
— joint stiffness
— joint pain
— cold intolerance
— bone pain or tenderness
— unusual or strange behaviour
— slow, sluggish, lethargic movement
— anxiety, stress, and tension
— groin lump
— generalised itching (pruritus)

— genital sores (female)
— genital sores (male)
— blurred vision
— double vision (diplopia)
— light sensitivity
— blind spots in the vision
— decreased vision or blindness
— chest pain
— flank pain or pain in the sides
— back pain
— abdominal pain
— loss of appetite, indigestion, or other gastrointestinal upset
— muscle pain
— bone pain or tenderness
— numbness and tingling
— seizures.

DIAGNOSIS

HIV infection is diagnosed on the basis of blood tests using three different ELISA/Rapid simple tests using different antigen preparation. AIDS cases are diagnosed on the basis of two different ELISA/Rapid tests on different antigens and presence of AIDS related opportunistic infections. Western Blot test is used for confirmation of diagnosis of indeterminate ELISA tests.

Development of characteristic infections and tumours, called opportunistic infections of AIDS and AIDS defining manifestations of immune deficiency, may occur. Sometimes the presence of one of these disorders is the first sign that AIDS is present.

i) HIV antibody test ELISA (Enzyme Linked Immuno-absorbent Assay) and western blot are positive

ii) absolute CD4 lymphocyte count is less than 200

iii) p24 antigen is abnormal

iv) T (thymus derived) lymphocyte count is abnormal.

TREATMENTS

There is no cure for AIDS at this time. However, treatments are available that can improve the quality of life of those suffering the infection.

i) Antiviral therapy suppresses the replication of the HIV infection in the body. Retrovir, also called Zidovudine or AZT, is an antiviral agent most frequently used in treatment for AIDS.

ii) Saquinavir, manufactured under the trade name Invirase, has recently been approved by the FDA for use in the treatment of AIDS. It is the first to be approved in a new group of drugs claimed to be 10 times stronger than existing anti-virals used in AIDS treatment.

iii) Other antiviral agents are in investigational stages. Hematopoietic stimulating factors are sometimes used to treat anaemia and low white blood cell counts associated with AIDS.

iv) Preventive measures to avoid opportunistic infections such as *Pneumocystis carinii pneumonia* is possible with medications and can keep AIDS patients healthier for longer periods of time. Opportunistic infections are treated as they occur.

v) The emotional stress of devastating illnesses can often be helped by joining support groups where members share common experiences and problems.

To avoid AIDS:

i) Use condoms
ii) Use of disposable syringes and needles
iii) Avoid multiple partners
iv) Use of HIV free blood
v) Proper treatment of sexually transmitted diseases.

HIV is not spread by:

i) Drinking water or eating food from the same utensils used by infected person
ii) Sharing toilets
iii) Shaking hands
iv) Hugging or kissing
v) Donating blood
vi) Working with people who are HIV infected
vii) Massage and rub each other's bodies
viii) Swimming in pools used by people with HIV/AIDS
ix) Through mosquito bite
x) Socialising or casually living with people with HIV/AIDS.

There are some other factors which also should taken into consideration to prevent the epidemic:

i) Blood products like plasma, Factor 8, Rh Factor, immunoglobulin, interferon, etc., also should not be accepted until one is sure that they have been screened for HIV.
ii) In case of requirement of blood always prefer to accept blood from family and friends instead of buying blood from professional donors as one cannot be sure of the quality of blood donated by him.

iii) Donating blood does not carry the risk of transmission of HIV infection as the needles used for these purposes are sterile.

iv) You could rule out the risk of acquiring HIV infection when you go in for a blood-test if the equipment being used on you is sterile.

v) Menstrual blood of an HIV positive woman is infective.

vi) Mosquitoes are not capable of transmitting HIV infection as the HIV is not able to survive or replicate inside the intestine of the mosquito.

vii) Medical personnel are at a potential risk of acquiring HIV infection as they have to deal with blood and other body risk is very minimal if precautionary measures such as use of gloves, masks and goggles, are taken when handling potentially infected material.

viii) Dried blood is not infective as the HIV cannot live long outside the body and cannot survive in a dried form.

AIDS: GLOBAL OVERVIEW

The scale of the AIDS crisis now outstrips even the worst-case scenarios of a decade ago. Dozens of countries are already in the grip of serious HIV/AIDS epidemics, and many more are on the brink. Around the world, an estimated five million people became infected in 2001, 800 000 of them children. Over the next decade, without effective treatment and care, they will join the ranks of the more-than 20 million people who have died of AIDS since the first clinical evidence of HIV/AIDS was in 1981. It is equally clear that the vast majority of people (including those living in countries with high national HIV prevalence) have not yet acquired the virus. Enabling them to protect themselves against HIV, and providing adequate and affordable treatment and care to people living with the virus, represent two of the biggest challenges facing humankind today.

Asia and the Pacific

Despite well-documented and successful HIV-prevention programmes in a few countries, the HIV/AIDS epidemic continues to spread in Asia and the Pacific. In the past two years, the situation has changed rapidly in several parts of the region. This region serves as a reminder that no country is immune to a serious HIV epidemic. Low national prevalence rates conceal serious, localised epidemics in several areas, including China and India, where large numbers of people are infected and affected proof that national HIV prevalence figures do not tell the full story of the epidemic. In fact, the region as a whole is home to more people living with HIV/AIDS than any other besides sub-Saharan Africa -an estimated 6.6 million people at the end of 2001, including the 1 million adults and children who were newly infected with HIV in that year. Less than 30 000 people are on anti-retroviral treatment in this region.

In China, home to a fifth of the world's people, HIV is moving into new groups of the population and raising the spectre of a much more widespread epidemic. Surveillance data on China's huge population are sketchy, but it is estimated that around 850 000 Chinese were living with HIV/AIDS in 2001, with HIV infections having risen more than 67 per cent in the first six months of 2001. Several HIV epidemics are being observed among certain population groups in different parts of this vast country. Serious localised HIV epidemics are occurring among injecting drug users in at least seven provinces. Another nine provinces are possibly on the brink of similar HIV epidemics because of very high rates of needle-sharing.

There are also signs of heterosexually transmitted HIV epidemics in at least three provinces. Widespread attention has been devoted to the serious epidemics in Henan Province in central China, where many tens of thousands (and possibly more) of rural villagers have become infected since the early 1990s by selling their blood to collecting centres that did not follow basic blood-donation safety procedures. There are concerns that similar tragedies might have unfolded in other provinces. Overall, it has been estimated that 150 000 (and possibly many more) people may have been infected through these practices.

Several other factors highlight the need for swift action if a much more serious epidemic is to be prevented. Sexually transmitted infections increased significantly from 430 000 cases in 1997 to 860 000 cases in 2000. This suggests that unprotected sex with non-monogamous partners is on the rise in China. Massive population mobility, and increasing socioeconomic disparities add to the likelihood of wider HIV spread.

By expanding prevention and care efforts across the entire nation, China can avert millions of HIV infections and save millions of lives in the coming decade. The five-year AIDS action plan promulgated in mid-2001 has signalled a strong commitment to take up the challenge. India, too, is experiencing serious, localised epidemics. At the end of 2001, India's national adult HIV prevalence rate was under 1 per cent, yet this meant that an estimated 3.97 million Indians were living with HIV/AIDS more than in any other country besides South Africa. The epidemic is spreading among the general population and beyond groups with high-risk behaviour. Indeed, median HIV prevalence among women attending antenatal clinics was higher than 2 per cent in Andhra Pradesh and exceeded 1 per cent in four other states (Karnataka, Maharashtra, Manipur and Tamil Nadu). India's epidemic is also strikingly diverse, both among and within states.

The factors facilitating the rapid spread of HIV/AIDS epidemics are present throughout the region. This is reflected in the fact that many countries are experiencing high HIV infection rates among some population groups mainly injecting drug users, sex workers and men who have sex with men. Across the region, injecting drug use offers the epidemic huge scope for growth. Upwards of 50 per cent of injecting drug users already have acquired the virus in Myanmar, Nepal, Thailand and Manipur in India. Recent surveys show very high rates of needle sharing among users in other countries, including Bangladesh and Viet Nam. It is vital that more effective HIV prevention programmes among injecting drug users be introduced.

Male-to-male sex occurs in all countries of the region and features significantly in the epidemic, despite much official denial. Countries that have measured HIV prevalence among men who have sex with men have found it to be high 14 per cent in Cambodia in 2000, for example, roughly the same level among Thai male sex workers, and up to 10 per cent in several states in Malaysia. Indonesia, the world's fourth most populous country, shows just how suddenly a HIV/AIDS epidemic can emerge. After more than a decade of negligible HIV prevalence rates, the country is now seeing infection rates increase rapidly among injecting drug users and sex workers, in some places, along with an exponential rise in infection among blood donors.

Although injecting drug use is a relatively recent phenomenon in this country, HIV prevalence measured in one drug treatment centre in the capital, Jakarta, rose from 15.4 per cent in 2000 to over 40 per cent by mid-2001. Among the Pacific Island countries and territories, Papua New Guinea has the highest HIV infection rates. Although prevalence of HIV is still low in the wider population, recent studies in the capital, Port Moresby, have found high HIV prevalence levels among female sex workers (17 per cent) and people attending sexually transmitted infection clinics (7 per cent in 1999). Given the very low levels of condom use, and very high rates of sexually transmitted infections, the country could see HIV spreading beyond these groups.

The Philippines, meanwhile, has taken strong action against HIV/AIDS. To date, this has helped keep HIV prevalence low, but there are risks that an epidemic could grow, especially if efforts are not quickly expanded. High rates of other sexually transmitted infections among Filipino sex workers, their clients and men who have sex with men indicate low levels of condom use. Fewer than half of sex workers in the Philippines using condoms with every client.

Thailand and Cambodia have shown that the 'natural' course of the epidemic can be changed. Early, large-scale prevention programmes, which include efforts directed at both those with higher risk behaviour and the broader population, can keep infection rates lower in specific groups and reduce the risk of extensive HIV spread in the wider population. In the past two years, Cambodia has demonstrated that consistent political commitment at all levels can bring the epidemic under control. HIV prevalence among pregnant women in major urban areas declined from 3.2 per cent in 1996 to 2.7 per cent at the end of 2000, thanks to a multifaceted response that includes a 100 per cent condom use programme, and steps to counter stigma and reduce people's vulnerability. In 2001, the country took another step forward by enacting a new and inclusive national AIDS strategic plan based on analysis undertaken by the Cambodian authorities.

HIV/AIDS has now been main-streamed into the strategic plans of several ministries, including the Ministry of National Defence. This allows Cambodia to expand successful projects nationally, and to tackle outstanding issues such as blood safety, which remains a major concern. Thailand, though, is also a reminder that success can be relative. Its well funded, politically supported and comprehensive prevention programmes have saved millions of lives, reducing the number of new HIV infections from 143 000 in 1991 to 29 000 in 2001. None the less, one in 100 Thais in this country of 63.6 million people are infected with HIV, and AIDS has become the leading cause of death. There is concern that, unless prevention efforts are adapted to changes in the epidemic, it could break out of its current pattern and spread further. At particular risk are the spouses of sex workers clients, young people, injecting drug users, men who have sex with men, and mobile populations.

Eastern Europe and Central Asia

HIV/AIDS is spreading rapidly through countries of this region, which continues to experience the fastest growing epidemic in the world. In 2001, there were an estimated 250 000 new infections, bringing to one million the number of people living with HIV/AIDS. Less than 1000 people are estimated to be receiving anti-retroviral treatment. Except for isolated epidemics in the early 1990s (related to injecting drug use in Poland, and to nosocomial infections among thousands of children in Romania), no country of the region was many HIV infections in 1994. This began to change with the first widespread outbreak of HIV in Ukraine and Belarus in 1995. The epidemic then started to take off in other countries of the region Moldova in 1996 and the Russian Federation in 1998, followed by Latvia and then Kazakhstan.

In the Russian Federation, the startling increase in HIV infections of recent years is continuing. Almost 83 000 new HIV positive diagnoses were in 2001, raising the total number of HIV infections since the epidemic began to more than 173 000 in 2001 up from the 10 993 at the end of 1998. The estimated number of people now living with HIV/AIDS in the Russian Federation is thought to be around four times higher than these figures. HIV incidence is rising sharply in other countries, too. In Estonia, infections have soared from 12 in 1999 to 1474 in 2001. The same pattern appears in Latvia, where infections rose from 25 in 1997 to 807 in 2001.

The epidemic is growing in Kazakhstan, where 1175 HIV infections were in 2001. Swift spread of HIV is now also evident in Azerbaijan, Georgia, Kyrgyzstan, Tajikistan and Uzbekistan. Ukraine, with an estimated adult HIV prevalence rate of 1 per cent, remains the most affected country in the region and, indeed, in all of Europe. An estimated 250 000 people were living with HIV in this country of nearly 50 million. While three-quarters of cumulative HIV infections in Ukraine are related to injecting drug use, the proportion of sexually transmitted HIV infections is increasing.

Although their absolute numbers remain small, more people (mostly women) appear to be contracting HIV through sexual transmission and more pregnant women are testing positive for HIV, suggesting a shift of the epidemic into the wider population. In the psychological and socioeconomic aftermath of the recent conflicts in the Balkans, young people have become more vulnerable to HIV. Currently, there is little evidence that the HIV/AIDS epidemic has become well established there, but limited surveillance data means that the actual levels or trends in the epidemic are not clear.

A recent, extensive rapid assessment study by WHO and UNICEF found high levels of drug injection in some places, along with frequent sharing of injecting equipment. Among men who have sex with men, and sex workers, condom use is low. The study also found strong overlap between these groups at higher risk. For example, in Serbia, 20 per cent of sex workers and 18 per cent of men who have sex with men were found to inject drugs. Several factors are creating a fertile setting for the epidemic.

The opening of borders has drawn several countries in the region into the globalised circuits of drug trafficking. Mass unemployment and economic insecurity be set much of the region. The rigid social control of the past has eroded, and new common norms and values are yet to become firmly grounded. Public health and other services are steadily deteriorating in some countries. Unprecedented numbers of young people do not complete their secondary schooling. In the Commonwealth of Independent States, the vast majority of HIV infections are among young people chiefly among those who inject drugs. It is estimated that up to 1 per cent of the population of those countries is injecting drugs, placing these people and their sexual partners at high risk of infection.

Sentinel surveillance in St. Petersburg in 2000, for example, revealed an increase in HIV prevalence from 12 per cent to 19. 3 per cent among injecting drug users in one year. There is evidence that young people in several countries are becoming sexually active at an earlier age and that premarital sex is increasing. A steady rise in premarital sex is being observed among Romanian adolescent girls (aged 15-19), for example. The percentage of premarital sexual relations in 1993 (9 per cent) had more than doubled to 22 per cent in 1999, while a 2000 in Ukraine found that about 51 per cent of women aged 15 -24 had a premarital sexual relationship.

In some Central Asian republics, as of 2001, awareness of HIV/AIDS was still dismal among vulnerable groups, such as adolescent (15 -19-year-old) girls a mere 10 per cent of whom in Tajikistan had ever heard of HIV/AIDS. In 2001, in Azerbaijan and Uzbekistan, fewer than 60 per cent were aware of the disease. The proportion of young girls harbouring at least one major misconception about HIV/AIDS ranged from 94 per cent to 98 per cent in those countries. In Ukraine, which has the highest HIV prevalence rate in Europe, only 9 per cent of adolescent girls were aware of HIV prevention methods. Although improving in some countries, levels of condom use remain low. In the 2000, Ukraine referred to earlier, only 28 per cent of the young women had used a condom when they first had sex. Meanwhile, very high rates of sexually transmitted infections continue to be found in Eastern Europe and Central Asia, compounding the odds of HIV being transmitted through unprotected sex.

In 2000, the number of newly cases of syphilis in the Russian Federation stood at 157 per 100 000 persons, compared to 4.2 per 100 000 persons in 1987. Similar general trends are visible in the other countries of the Commonwealth of Independent States, in the Baltic States and in Romania. HIV risk is also high among men who have sex with men, among whom multiple partners and unprotected sex are widespread. While laws penalising homosexual activities with imprisonment have been struck off the statute-books in most countries of the former Soviet Union, this group remains highly stigmatised socially. Recently, gay groups have started HIV prevention activities for men who have sex with men in

Belarus, Ukraine and several Central Asian republics. Overall, though, coverage remains minimal.

Central Europe offers cause for moderate optimism. By mounting a strong national response, the Polish Government has successfully curtailed the epidemic among injecting drug users and prevented it from gaining a foothold in the wider population. Prevalence remains low in countries such as the Czech Republic, Hungary and Slovenia, where well-designed national HIV/AIDS programmes are in operation. There are other signs of growing political commitment in the region. Members of the Commonwealth of Independent States were the first to organise a regional follow-up to the 2001 United Nations General Assembly Special Session on HIV/AIDS, and recently endorsed a regional Programme of Work on HIV/AIDS.

In countries such as Bulgaria, Romania, the Russian Federation and Ukraine, the budgets of national AIDS programmes have increased considerably. Stronger partnerships are also being forged between governments, the private sector and non-governmental organisations, with Ukraine setting a strong example on this front. Despite the economic hardships and public spending cuts that are weakening many countries health systems and general infrastructure, the capacity of the region remains generally good. This is particularly true for human resources. People are generally well educated, and the illiteracy rate remains low.

Many countries have managed to adopt best practices, and considerable efforts are being made in training and capacity-building in prevention and care. For many, too, national strategic plans on HIV/AIDS, which identify young people and vulnerable groups as priorities, have been developed. More than 150 HIV/AIDS prevention projects among injecting drug users now operate across the region, along with projects focusing on other vulnerable populations such as prison inmates, sex workers and men who have sex with men. Building on these achievements, the current challenge is to expand coverage, develop and implement more comprehensive approaches to reduce vulnerability among young people, and create better access to care for those who are becoming ill.

STRUGGLE AGAINST AIDS

In the past two years, the sense of common purpose in the worldwide struggle against HIV/AIDS has intensified. More than at any other time in the short history of the epidemic, the need to translate local and national examples of success into a global movement has become manifest. The political momentum to tackle AIDS has grown. Public opinion in many countries has been mobilised by the media, non-governmental organisations, activists, doctors, economists, and people living with HIV/AIDS. Communities and nations are progressively taking the lead in responding to the epidemic with increased political commitment, resources and institutional initiatives. But this new political resolve is not universal. An unacceptable number of governments and civil society institutions are still in a state of denial about the HIV/AIDS epidemic, and are failing to act to prevent its further spread or alleviate its impact. By failing to act, governments and civil society are turning their backs on the possibility of success against AIDS.

Where the moment of action has been seized, there is mounting evidence of inroads being made against the epidemic. Alongside the familiar achievements of Senegal, Thailand and Uganda, there are new successes on every continent. Despite emerging from genocide and conflict, Cambodia responded to the threat of HIV in the mid-1990s and has achieved marked declines in both the levels of HIV and the high-risk behaviours associated with its transmission. The infection rate among pregnant women in Cambodia declined by almost a third between 1997 and 2000. The Philippines has acted early to forestall the epidemic, keeping HIV rates low with strong prevention efforts and the mobilisation of community and business organisations. Brazil remains a leading example of the integration of comprehensive care and a renewed commitment to prevention.

The numbers of new HIV infections have been kept much lower than forecast less than a decade ago, while the 1996 decision to establish a legal right to free medication has brought treatment and care to more than 100 000 HIV-positive people. As a result, the number of annual AIDS deaths in Brazil in 2000 was a third of that in 2000. The annual cost of medication is more than outweighed by the resulting health-care and related savings. Similar legislation-led drug-access models are being pursued across Central and South America. In Africa, Zambia's focus on HIV prevention among youth and its efforts to involve businesses farmers, schools and religious groups in the fight against AIDS are proving successful.

The proportion of pregnant urban women aged 15 -19 who were HIV-positive had fallen from 28.4 per cent in 1993 to less than 14.8 per cent five years later. Examples of success come both from settings where HIV prevalence is low and from those where the impact of HIV/AIDS is already substantial. Both environments present challenges. Even where rapid increases in the epidemic are evident, yet population-wide prevalence is low, it is all too easy to marginalise HIV.

Growing political engagement in the response to AIDS is grounded in two decades of AIDS activism, led by individuals and communities whose lives have been touched by the epidemic. Organisations as diverse as the Gay Men's Health Crisis in New York, The AIDS Support Organisation in Uganda, the Save Your Generation Association in Ethiopia, Grupo Pela Vidda in Rio de Janeiro, and many hundreds of others like them, are built on the same foundations: an initially small group of people responding to the impact of AIDS by coming together to provide mutual support and take action. An activist movement responding to AIDS now exists globally. It has many aspects: community groups providing home-based care, treatment activists working through media and the law courts to extend access to HIV drugs, networks such as the International Council of AIDS Service Organisations and its regional bodies, and associations of HIV-positive people nationally and internationally, together with positive women's networks.

The presence of non-governmental and community-based organisations was notable at the United Nations General Assembly Special Session on HIV/AIDS in June 2001, providing a sense of urgency and conscience to Member State deliberations. The Global Fund to Fight AIDS, Tuberculosis and Malaria has modelled a new way of working by including on its Board not only non-governmental organisation representatives but also a seat for people who are themselves directly affected. The bedrock of activism, sustained in communities motivated to take action against AIDS, is key in driving political momentum locally, nationally and globally.

In April 2001, at the African Summit on HIV/AIDS, Tuberculosis and Other Related Infectious Diseases, in Abuja, Nigeria, UN Secretary General Kofi Annan issued a global call to action in the fight against AIDS. The personal priority he has given to AIDS has helped energise the United Nations system, as well as engage political and business leaders in the challenge. At the Millennium Summit of the United Nations in September 2000, 43 Heads of State and Government from both countries heavily affected and those less so, referred to AIDS as one of the most pressing problems worldwide. Presidents and prime ministers, particularly those from Africa and the Caribbean, but also those in Asia and Western and Eastern Europe, are displaying a personal commitment to the fight against AIDS. AIDS is now a prominent issue at international gatherings North and South. It has been on the agenda of summits and decision-making forums of the G8 and G77 nations, the Organisation of American States, the Organisation of African Unity, the Commonwealth of Nations, the European Union, the Association of South-East Asian Nations, and the Caribbean Community Secretariat (CARICOM). Both the World Economic Forum and the World Social Forum (in Porto Alegre) have held key sessions on AIDS and its global implications. The UN Security Council held its first-ever debate on AIDS in January 2000 the first time it had examined a health or development issue. Since then, it has held two more public debates on AIDS.

The new political momentum culminated in June 2001 when the membership of the United Nations met in a Special Session of the General Assembly to agree on a comprehensive and coordinated global response to the AIDS crisis. The members adopted a powerful Declaration of Commitment, and reaffirmed the pledge (made by world leaders in their Millennium Declaration) to halt and begin to reverse the spread of AIDS by 2015. The UN General Assembly Special Session on HIV/AIDS differed from the hundreds of meetings and summits held on AIDS in the past 20 years in this crucial respect: it was a meeting of all States, acting as governments. As such, it yielded both a common mandate and a basis for political accountability. The Special Session's Declaration of Commitment, adopted unanimously, now serves as a benchmark for global action. Its targets and goals include the need to:

i) secure more resources to fight AIDS, increasing annual spending to US$7-10 billion in low-and middle-income countries;

ii) ensure, by 2005, that a wide range of prevention programmes are available in all countries;

iii) by 2005, to ensure that at least 90 per cent of young people aged 15 -24 have access to information, education and services necessary to develop the life skills needed to reduce their vulnerability to HIV, and 95 per cent by 2010;

iv) reduce by 25 per cent the rate of HIV infection among young people aged 15-24 in the most affected countries by 2005 and globally by 2010;

v) reduce by 20 per cent by 2005 and 50 per cent by 2010 the proportion of infants born with HIV;

vi) by 2003, enact or strengthen anti-discrimination and human rights protections for people living with HIV/AIDS and for vulnerable groups;

vii) by 2003, develop or strengthen participatory programmes to protect the health of those most affected by HIV/AIDS;

viii) empower women as an essential part of reducing vulnerability to HIV;

ix) by 2003, develop national strategies to strengthen health-care systems and address factors affecting the provision of HIV-related drugs, including affordability and pricing; and

x) make treatment and care for people with HIV/AIDS as fundamental to the AIDS response as is prevention.

The Special Session on HIV/AIDS revealed continuing differences between States on how to respond to marginalised groups, such as men who have sex with men, injecting drug users and sex workers. Nevertheless, the Declaration expressed unanimous approval of fundamental approaches to tackling the epidemic, based on frank and forthright responses grounded in respect for human rights. The Declaration of Commitment provides the world with a basis for effective political action and a yardstick of accountability. At international, regional and national gatherings since the Special Session, the Declaration of Commitment has served to define agendas and create a common platform for action. Within weeks of the Special Session, implementation of the Declaration of Commitment was receiving regional attention.

Underpinning the renewed global resolve in tackling AIDS is a series of shifts in fundamental thinking about the epidemic.

i) We now realise that the HIV/AIDS epidemic is at an early stage of development and that its long-term evolution is still unclear. Despite the epidemic's manifest potential for explosive growth within a matter of years, its overall dynamic needs to be considered in a timeframe of decades.

ii) Successful, proven approaches to HIV prevention have been identified, and the need for a particular emphasis on young people has been recognised. In every country where HIV transmission has been reduced, it has been among young people (and with their determination) that the most spectacular reductions have occurred.

iii) Community mobilisation is the core strategy on which success against HIV has been built. Fostering such mobilisation requires eliminating stigma, developing partnerships between social and government actors, and systematically involving communities and individuals infected and affected by HIV/AIDS.

iv) Access to comprehensive care and treatment for HIV/AIDS is not an optional luxury in global responses. Access to care is a basic necessity in programming in every setting — from the wealthiest to the poorest — and needs to encompass the full continuum, including home-based and palliative care, treatment of opportunistic infections and anti-retroviral therapy.

Responding to demands for more equitable access to care is integral to creating broad, demand-driven strategies that respond to the desire by households and communities to protect themselves from HIV and its effects.

The Millennium Development Goals, arising from the UN Millennium Summit of September 2000, include a commitment to halt and begin to reverse the global spread of AIDS by 2015. They also include the following goals: to halve global poverty; ensure primary-school education for all; promote gender equality and empower women; and reduce child mortality while improving maternal health. This total package is integral to success in alleviating the impact of AIDS. Finally, lack of capacity to absorb increased resources allocated for HIV/AIDS, while posing challenges, is no reason to delay the boosting of responses in countries expressing commitment to an expanded response. Assessments of programme readiness carried out by UNAIDS, together with rapid responses to calls for proposals from the new Global Fund to Fight AIDS, Tuberculosis and Malaria, are both demonstrations of immediate and substantial unmet needs in AIDS programming in much of the world.

Partnerships are emerging in response to AIDS, with increased involvement across the whole of government as well as between governments, civil society and the business sector. Trade unions and women's and youth organisations are engaging in AIDS-related activities, often for the first time. Business coalitions on AIDS have spread, especially in Asia and Africa. Globally, businesses have recognised the need for a proactive AIDS agenda, and efforts in this direction are being spearheaded by the Global Business Council on AIDS. The International Labour Organisation (ILO) became UNAIDS eighth Cosponsor in 2001. It has engineered a new code of conduct designed to protect and support workers with HIV/ AIDS and to use workplaces more effectively in the fight against AIDS.

The World Food Programme is lending its support to AIDS responses in its field of operations, while the International Federation of Red Cross and Red Crescent Societies has begun to tackle AIDS-related stigma, starting with its workers and volunteers. The new paradigm in access to care is beginning to take effect, and long-standing global inequities are being challenged. From disputes before the World Trade Organisation, to court cases in South Africa, debate in relation to essential medicines has been resolved in favour of lowering trade barriers to access.

The principle of preferential pricing for HIV drugs for low and middle income countries has been largely accepted in the pharmaceutical industry. Prices have begun to drop and countries rights to invoke compulsory or voluntary licensing arrangements on patented drugs and medications were affirmed clearly at the World Trade Organisation meeting in Doha, Qatar, in late 2001. Generic versions of many anti-retroviral drugs now exist.

Important progress has been made in the prevention of mother-to-child transmission. New guidelines on anti-retro-viral therapy and infant-feeding for HIV-infected mothers have been developed. Voluntary counselling and testing need to go beyond the 1 per cent of women in sub-Saharan Africa currently being reached. Antenatal care infrastructure has to expand. And safe infant-feeding by HIV-infected mothers must become an actual choice, rather than a theoretical one. Much work remains to be done, however, in transforming the successes of small pilot projects into large-scale programmes. As with the epidemic in general, access to HIV treatment also has governance and security dimensions. Even in the poorest countries, in urban areas, in particular, there is already a huge backlog in demand for HIV treatment.

Huge global challenges still shape the context in which the world confronts the epidemic. Failure to control AIDS is an index of inequitable development and poor governance. Income inequality, gender inequality, labour migration, conflict and refugee movement all promote the spread of HIV. Despite the widely recognised benefits of globalisation, more than a billion of the world's six billion people still cannot fulfil their basic needs for food, water, sanitation, health care, housing and education. Worldwide, an estimated 1.1 billion people are malnourished. In more than 30 of the poorest national economies, real per capita incomes have been declining since the early 1980s. At the same time, pressures on States to provide basic services and infrastructure have not eased.

The HIV/AIDS epidemic, along with other diseases, conflicts and droughts, is worsening matters further. But the global response to AIDS shows that the negative effects of globalisation need not be 'facts of life'. Greater access to high-income countries markets, debt relief and more development aid will go a long way towards enabling countries to reduce poverty. High income countries spent more than US$300 billion in 2001 on agricultural subsidies—roughly equivalent to the combined gross domestic product of all of sub-Saharan Africa. It is clear that AIDS represents a long and devastating tale of exclusion for millions of people, with or without HIV infection. The expanding AIDS epidemic provides a compelling case for accelerating much-needed global reform in an effort to better support local responses. This can be done by:

i) creating stronger international cooperation, guided by the principles of human rights;

ii) generating more accountability and transparency of international institutions;

iii) replenishing national capabilities to safeguard the right to health and enlisting the help of the business sector in such efforts;

iv) redressing global poverty by, among other things, increasing Official Development Assistance to at least 0.7 per cent of gross national product.

The world cannot afford to wait until the perfect conditions exist before acting against AIDS. The fight against AIDS cannot go on hold until human security is achieved and poverty is eliminated. The growing global response to AIDS needs to be bolstered by stronger human security, equality and justice. In the long run, success in the struggle against the epidemic requires a global community that acts on the basis of human concern and humane values.

REFERENCES

Cockerell, C. J., Cutaneous and historic signs of HIV infection other than Kaposi's sarcoma. In G. P. Wormser (ed.), *AIDS and other manifestations of HIV infection,* New York: Raven Press, 1992.

Finley, J. L., Joshi, V. V., & Neil, J. S. A., General pathology of HIV infection. In G. P. Wormser (ed.)*AIDS and other manifestations of HIV infection.* New York: Raven Press, 1992.

Fischl, M. A., Treatment of HIV infection, In M. A. Sande & P. A. Volberding (eds.), *The medical management of AIDS.* Philadelphia: Saunders, 1992.

Gordon, G., and T. Klouda, *Preventing a Crisis: AIDS and Family Planning Work:* London: International Planned Parenthood Federation, 1989.

Sierra Health Foundation, *Challenge for the future: Coordinating HIV/AIDS care and services in the next decade.* Rancho Cordova, 1991.

UNAIDS Report on the Global HIV/AIDS Epidemic, 2002.

2

HIV/AIDS in South Asia

South Asia has 4.2 million people living with HIV/AIDS, equivalent to a prevalence rate below 1 per cent of the adult population. However, the relatively low prevalence disguises the presence of high risk factors which continues to make HIV/AIDS as significant challenge to development. HIV infection has taken root in South Asia, and poses a threat to development and poverty alleviation efforts in the region. The trend of increasing HIV infections, combined with heightened social and economic vulnerabilities that are fuelled by extensive commercial sex, injecting drug use, low condom use and access, and population movements highlights the need to act quickly and effectively. Unless actions are now taken to scale up the response to curb the spread of HIV/AIDS, it could lead to significant economic and social consequences for all sectors. Because HIV/AIDS is not solely a health issue, an effective response requires a multi-sectoral partnership. Responding to HIV/AIDS now would cost only a fraction of what will be required at a later stage when the disease is allowed to become more widespread.

While overall prevalence rates remain relatively low, South Asia has about 5 million HIV-infected persons of the world's 34 million people living with HIV/AIDS. The region has large populations. Thus, a rise of a mere 0.1 percent in prevalence rate, for example in India, would increase the national total of adults living with HIV by over a half million persons. According to the Indian National AIDS Control Organisation, about 4 million Indians are already infected, and the number of new infections is expected to double every 14 months. This makes India, along with South Africa, the country with the largest absolute number of HIV-infected in the world. Nepal has a concentrated epidemic, characterised by a low prevalence rate among the general population but significantly higher rates among high-risk behaviour groups, such as injecting drug users and sex workers. For example, about 45 per cent of the injecting drug using population in Katmandu is infected with HIV.

Bangladesh, Pakistan, and Sri Lanka have nascent epidemics, and the threat of HIV spread is significant because of high prevalence of risk behaviours and high vulnerability. Bhutan and the Maldives also have nascent epidemics, but with a relatively moderate level of risk.

A number of factors have played a significant role in the spread of HIV in Asia and are likely to continue having an impact: injecting drug use, commercial sex, literacy, dependency, access to information and services, migration and population mobility. While the prevalence rates among adults aged 15 to 49 in most countries in Asia and the Pacific is below one percent (higher only in Cambodia, Myanmar and Thailand) within particular populations or geographic areas the virus is exacting a terrible toll. For this reason it can be misleading to focus solely on prevalence rates in general populations.

In Malaysia, Nepal, Vietnam and some provinces of China the rates of infection among injecting drug users is extremely high. According to some estimates, there are 3 million drug users in China. Needle sharing appears common, with more than 45 percent of injectors sharing needles. HIV infection is reported among injecting drug users from 25 provinces. In both China and Vietnam 65 to 70 percent of detected HIV infections have been among injectors.

China and India between them account for around 36 percent of the world's population. With such huge populations, even low HIV prevalence rates translate into huge numbers of infections. In India, 3.7 million people were living with HIV/

AIDS at the beginning of the millennium more than in any other country in the world except South Africa. In both China and India, the epidemic varies widely from region to region, both in size and in method of transmission. With 100 million people or more on the move, China is experiencing population movement that dwarfs any other in recorded history. In addition, having practically eradicated sexually transmitted infections by the 1960s, China is now seeing a steep rise in these rates over the last several years. Reported cases increased from 5,800 in 1985 to over 836,000 in 1999.

In parts of northeast India, widespread injecting drug use has provided an early entry point for HIV. In Manipur, the prevalence of HIV infection among injecting drug users shot up from virtually nothing in 1988 to over 70 percent just four years later. It has remained at these high levels ever since. Around 2.2 percent of pregnant women in Manipur tested positive for HIV in 1999. In other states, even higher levels of HIV have been recorded among pregnant women. Most cases of infection appear to have been acquired from husbands who had been infected in turn by sex workers, themselves part of a longer chain of transmission. By the mid-1990s, a quarter or more of sex workers in cities such as New Delhi, Hyderabad, Madurai, Pune, Tirupati and Vellore tested positive for HIV. In Mumbai, the prevalence of HIV infection among sex workers reached 71 percent in 1997. In other parts of the country, there is evidence that unsafe sex is spreading HIV within the general population.

In most Southeast Asian countries, HIV was not diagnosed until 1984 or later. In this region the first patient with AIDS was reported in 1984 from Thailand. Since then, however, HIV infection has spread extremely rapidly and WHO estimates that currently there are 5 million HIV-infected people in the region, which is 18 per cent of the global total. Besides persons with high risk behaviours, HIV infection rates have now begun to increase in general population as well.

Since the beginning of the epidemic, a total of 151,804 cases of AIDS have been diagnosed and reported in the region - more than 48 per cent increase from 65,091 cases reported upto 1 July 1997. Thailand, India and Myanmar continue to report the largest number of cases – 135,950, 12,239 and 2,854 respectively — accounting for more than 95 per cent of the cases reported from the Region to date.

Although Bhutan has diagnosed persons with HIV infection, so far only one case has been reported and DPR Korea have not yet reported AIDS cases. Allowing the under-diagnosis, incomplete reporting and reporting delay, and based on the available data on HIV infections around the world, it is estimated that less than 25 per cent of the total AIDS have been reported. Analysis of recent data show that 91 per cent were between the ages of 15-49 years and 4.6 per cent were children; male to female ratio was 4:1. Heterosexual intercourse was the most predominant mode of spread (85 per cent), followed by injecting drug use (7 per cent) and from mother to child (5 per cent).

HIV prevalence studies confirm the alarming increase in HIV infection rates in selected high-risk populations. In Thailand, HIV rates of 0 to less than 1 per cent among injecting drug-users (IDU) in Bangkok were found in various *ad hoc* surveys from 1985 to 1987. However, HIV rates increased sharply to 40 per cent by September 1988 and has now stabilised almost at that level. Rates similar to Bangkok were also seen in various other provinces around the country. This wave of HIV epidemic in IDU was followed by that among female prostitutes and, by successive waves of transmission, to male clients of the prostitutes, and from them to the wives and girl friends of these men in the general population. Recently, the prevalence rates were 34 per cent in IDUs, 27 per cent in low-charge prostitutes, 8.5 per cent in male STD patients and 1.8 per cent among pregnant women. Northern provinces are most severely affected. The national efforts, however, are now having an impact; the HIV infection rates among army conscripts have steady fallen from 4 per cent in 1993 to 2.1 per cent in 1995 and the number of STDs reported nationally have also declined to the record low levels.

Table 1

AIDS and HIV infections in South Asia as of September 2000

Country	*Report AIDS cases*	*Date of last report*	*Estimated HIV infections*	*Rates 100,000 population*
Bangladesh	12	06/99	21,000	16
Bhutan	1	08/98	<100	<16
India	12,239	06/2000	3,500,000	418
Maldives	5	06/99	<100	<25
Nepal	383	08/2000	25,000	66
Pakistan	NA	NA	NA	
Sri Lakna	105	06/99	7,500	32

In Manipur, North-East India, the epidemic which was mainly confined to injecting drug users, is now spreading into general population. None of the 2,322 IDUs seen from 1986 to 1989 were seropositive for HIV. However, the rate increased to 54 per cent during the period October 1989 to June 1990, and at present it is 77 per cent. In Bombay, the HIV seropositivity rates among prostitutes and STD patients are now 51 per cent and 35 per cent respectively. The rate among sex workers in Tamil Nadu in 1996 was 30 per cent. There is evidence of increase in HIV among women attending antenatal clinics; the seroprevalance in Bombay and Manipur during 1995 were 2.5 and 1 per cent respectively.

The most recent survey in an antenatal clinic in Bombay showed a HIV infection rate of 4.2 per cent. Similar explosive increases in HIV seropositivity have been documented in Myanmar too. As of March 1998, sentinel surveillance data show median rates among IDUs of 47 per cent, in male STD patients (5 per cent), CSWs (26 per cent) and pregnant women (2 per cent). Highest rates among IDU was seen in Mandalay (80 per cent) and among pregnant women in Taunggyi and Tachilek (5 per cent each). In some areas, HIV seroprevalence among samples of pregnant women has already reached 4-7 per cent level. Overall it appears that HIV infection rates nationally among IDUs have declined from 73 per cent in 1992 to 47 per cent in 1998.

There is every possibility of a similar scenario being repeated in other countries of the Region. Risk behaviours which promote the spread of HIV, such as injection of drugs, male patronage of prostitutes, high rates of STD and low condom usage, are present in all countries. In Nepal, for example, the HIV infection rates among sex workers and STD patients although very low, but doubled between 1992 and 1993. The prevalence in IDU has recently been reported to have increased sharply to 40 per cent. In Indonesia, HIV remains low in general but potential for spread can be indicated by outbreaks seen in Merauke and Maluku islands recently where a relatively high HIV infection rates was noted among various population groups such as blood donors and sex workers respectively.

Heterosexual contact is the predominant mode of HIV transmission in the region, that the rates of STD are high and that there is considerable unprotected sexual activity, continued transmission of HIV in the general population appears inevitable, unless effective measures are taken now in all countries! Predictions about AIDS tend to be unrealistic, but the current estimate of more than 5 million HIV infections in South-East Asia is nearly 18 per cent of the global total, while the proportion of reported AIDS cases is less than 6 per cent.

Wile the annual number of HIV infections will peak in Africa by 1995, infections in Asia will continue to increase well into the early next century. By the year 2000, the cumulative number of infection would be 8-10 million and the annual numbers would far exceed that seen in sub-Saharan Africa. Given the mean progression time for initial HIV infection to develop into AIDS, it can be concluded that AIDS cases in the Region will continue to increase well into the next century, and up to 2 million cumulative cases of AIDS may occur by the year 2000. These incidence estimates and projections are, however, contingent upon the effectiveness of current and future prevention efforts. Nonetheless, the annual toll of AIDS cases will continue to grow in the future, requiring further prevention efforts and increased medical and social services for the next several years for persons with HIV infection. In the wake of HIV pandemic, tuberculosis is beginning to increase in parts of Thailand and India.

The greatest tragedy, besides medical and health care costs, will be the loss of thousands of lives, particularly among young adults in their most productive age and infants born to HIV-infected mothers, directly affecting child survival rates. This will result in a major impact on the economy of all countries throughout the Region — in terms of direct medical and patient care costs and indirect costs in the form of absenteeism and decreased productivity.

Table 2

Adult HIV prevalence rates and estimated number of persons with HIV

	Adult HIV prevalence rates in percentage	Estimated persons with HIV
India	1 % Increasing, but with regional variation	4,000,000
Pakistan	0.1 % Up to 11 % among injecting drug users	75,000
Nepal	0.02 % 50 % among injecting drug users in Kathmandu	34,000
Bangladesh	< 0.03 % Up to 3 % among high risk groups	21,000
Sri Lanka	0.07 %	8,500
Maldives	0.05 %	65
Bhutan	Unknown	Few cases reported

Table 3
HIV/AIDS risk factors in South Asia

Risks	*Examples*
Commercial sex business &	There are an estimated 2,000,000 commercial sex workers (CSW) in India, 60% of them are in Mumbai, India who are HIV positive.
Low condom use	About 100,000 Nepali girls working in Indian brothels and an estimated 5,000-7,000 Nepali girls trafficked annually to India.
	Condom use among Bangladesh's 36,000 CSWs varies between 4- 28%.
Injecting drug use	Between 60,000–100,000 injecting drug users (IDUs) are in Pakistan and an estimated 20,000 IDUs in Nepal. There is a 50% HIV prevalence rate among IDUs in Kathmandu.
Low awareness	Over 95% of 15-19 year old Bangladeshis don't know a single method of HIV prevention. A 1999 Sri Lanka study among 9th grade students found that 63% could not name a single mode of HIV transmission and 75% could not identify a single method of HIV prevention.
Lack of blood safety	There is widespread use of unsterilized needles in Pakistan and exposure to infected blood or blood products accounts for approxi-mately 20% of repo-rted cases. 94% of injections are administered using reused injection equipment.
Extensive poverty High mobility	Many migrants are known to buy sex but do not have access to information, condoms or supportive services that would enable them to have safe sex.
Low status of women Trafficking of women	Gender inequality manifested by low social status, illiteracy, and lack of empowerment puts women at greater risk of HIV infection.
Illiteracy	Literacy rates vary widely between countries: in Nepal over 77% of women are illiterate, while only 3.6% of women in Maldives are illiterate. Regional illiteracy rates are 35% for men and 59% for women.

In the countries of the region, the pandemic is likely to overstretch an already fragile health and economic infrastructure. Some estimates indicate that the direct and the indirect cost of the pandemic by the year 2000 for Thailand and India would be US$ 9 billion and 11 billion respectively. The widespread presence of risk factors places the region under great threat. However, the HIV epidemics in most South Asian countries are still limited, thus providing windows of opportunities for timely preventive responses that are cost-effective.

REGIONAL HIV/AIDS STRATEGY

The South Asia region supports and promotes country-specific approaches which focus on preventing the further spread of HIV/AIDS in high risk populations, people in risk situations, youth, and in the general population. This regional strategy encourages a shift from a health-based approach to a broad-based strategy, specifically seeking to:

i) promote political commitment at all levels and in multiple sectors in order to create a supportive environment and actions for effective HIV/AIDS responses;

ii) encourage the inclusion of HIV/AIDS issues and programmes in the broader development agenda. Within a multi-sectoral framework, our development assistance is utilised through various channels, including government agencies, civil society organisations, non-governmental organisations, and the private sector.

iii) advance strategies that enhance community participation and community-based interventions and enable open discussions about HIV/AIDS, reduce stigma, and help prevent discrimination.

iv) emphasise the need for strengthened institutional capacity and the prioritisation of control efforts in areas where HIV programmes are still nascent.

Table 4

Goal and objectives HIV prevention strategies

Goal	Objectives	Main Programme/Projects Components
Reduce and prevent morbidity, mortality, and impact of AIDS	Reduce the rate of growth of HIV infection and prevent its spread	Targeted interventions for risk groups
		Preventive interventions for the general community and people in risk situations
		Promoting awareness
		Promoting community mobilization and participation
		Reducing stigma and discrimination
		Improving blood safety and rational use
		Controlling sexually transmitted diseases
		Treating opportunistic infections
		Developing clinical skills for AIDS care
		Promoting low-cost care and home care
	Strengthen the countries' capacity to respond to HIV/AIDS	Generating political commitment
		Planning sustainable programs and resource allocations
		Institutional strengthening
		Developing program management
		Enhancing skills
		Building surveillance and monitoring
		Intersectoral collaboration

Table 5
Current Indicative Level of Risks and Country Responses

Country	Level of vulnerability	Level of response
India		
(Federal level)	Very high	High
(State level)	Very high	Mixed among the states, ranging from high to low responses
Nepal	Very high	Low
Bangladesh	High	Medium
Pakistan	High	Low, being expanded
Sri Lanka	High	Low, being expanded
Maldives	Medium to High	Low
Bhutan	Medium to High	Medium
Afghanistan	High	Very low

REGIONAL RESPONSES

i) Co-sponsoring the Joint United Nations Programme on HIV/AIDS (UNAIDS).

ii) Strengthening institutional dialogue and partnership with UN agencies, bilaterals, NGOs, academic institutions, and global initiatives, including vaccine development.

iii) Promoting political will and commitment and ethical considerations to address the HIV/AIDS epidemic.

iv) Facilitating dialogue between countries to share lessons learned and good practices of intervention strategies and research.

v) Supporting cross-country collaboration to tackle cross-border issues, such as migration and trafficking.

vi) Development of a critical mass of technical skills in the Bank's South Asia Region to promote and support HIV/AIDS prevention and control efforts.

The current aggregate IDA-assisted Programmes/Projects and commitments for HIV/AIDS in South Asia amounts to about US$ 326.7 million.

Non-lending activities in South Asia largely involve policy and strategy dialogue, technical and economic advice, and advocacy to spur countries to act promptly and effectively against the threat of HIV. Other non-lending activities in the region have included assisting countries develop strategies for tackling HIV, as well as mobilising technical advisory services, which focus on capacity building and training, and sharing of knowledge, best practices, and lessons learned.

NATIONAL RESPONSES

While the AIDS epidemic continues to grow in the region, all countries are responding to this threat with urgency. The national AIDS programmes have developed strategic plans and implementing activities in partnership with various relevant sectors including NGOs and private sector. As a result, there are now a number of excellent examples which show that good progress is being made in responding to the pandemic in South-East Asia. Some examples are as follows:

The 100 per cent condom use programme in Thailand has received worldwide attention and can be considered as one of the most widely written and talked about programmes. The effectiveness of this programme can be assessed by the declining HIV incidence among military transcripts from 3.6 per cent in 1993 to 2.1 per cent in 1995.

The Sonagachi project in Calcutta, India, is another success story. The project, besides peer education, includes many other initiatives, such as provision of health care; literacy programme for peer educators, and schooling for children of sex workers. The project is a model for successful peer education programme among sex workers. The latest data show that HIV prevalence continues to be low — around 1.4 per cent, and that STDs are declining.

The interventions among injecting drug users (IDUs), including the needle exchange programme are being implemented successfully in Nepal. In Myanmar, the IEC and community-based treatment approach have been effective. As a result, the behavioural change is occurring among IDUs and HIV infection rates have come down to nearly 50 per cent from 66-73 per cent reported prior to 1994.

To prevent STDs, which is a huge burden in the Region, all the countries have now adopted the syndromic approach for STD case management. The integration of STD care into the general health services is now considered a major priority in the Region, and for this, the training of the primary health care workers and private practitioners is considered extremely important.

Although STD/AIDS prevention and control presents a daunting task ahead, the approaches adopted by the countries have been appropriate, relevant and effective. However, concerted and sustained efforts are needed in the future to combat the HIV/AIDS pandemic.

WHO SUPPORT

The role of WHO regarding HIV/AIDS vis-a-vis the new Joint and Co-sponsored UN Programme on HIV/AIDS (UNAIDS), which became operational on 1 January 1996, remains crucial. Given the country needs for support at this critical juncture in their fight against AIDS, WHO continues to provide technical, material and logistical support to national STD/AIDS prevention and control programmes in areas of its comparative advantage.

In Southeast Asia, this support will be provided by staff based in the WHO Regional Office in New Delhi as well as in selected countries, and in collaboration with other relevant WHO units/programmes and country offices. The SEARO STD/

AIDS Programme, while continuing to assist Member Countries, fully cooperates with UNAIDS as a co-sponsor of the Programme, particularly in health-related areas.

The objectives of the Regional STD/AIDS Programme are to:

i) Provide technical and programmatic support to Member States in the areas of HIV/AIDS and STD prevention and care;
ii) Support the WHO country offices in responding to the technical and operational needs of Member States, particularly of Ministries of Health;
iii) Assist other technical units in SEARO to mainstream/ incorporate HIV/AIDS into their existing programmes and activities, and
iv) Collaborate as one of the co-sponsors, with UNAIDS, in carrying out inter-country and regional activities in selected areas and programmes.

The WHO STD/AIDS Programme works within the framework of policies as accepted by the World Health Assembly meetings and articulated in the WHO Global AIDS Strategy Document, 1992. Further guidance on technical and programme matters are obtained from the WHO Strategic Plan, December 1996, and activities carried out in collaboration with UNAIDS and other co-sponsors. The priority strategies and interventions for support to governments in which WHO Regional Office takes a lead role, include:

i) Preventing HIV transmission by strengthening the STD case management capacities and health education activities
ii) Ensuring safe blood transfusions
iii) Providing comprehensive care to people infected with HIV or those with AIDS

iv) Monitoring the trends of the HIV/AIDS pandemic through surveillance, and supporting the HIV and STD-related research activities

v) Strengthening of laboratory services for STD and HIV/AIDS diagnosis

vi) Training of health care workers on STD/HIV/AIDS management.

The WHO continues to participate, along with other co-sponsors and UNAIDS, in the STD/AIDS programme planning, monitoring and evaluation missions to countries, as well as in advocacy activities. It actively promotes and facilitates the exchange/sharing of technical information and collaboration with all interested agencies.

Over the years, WHO staff and consultants have participated in the review of many national AIDS control programmes which resulted in specific recommendations for further strengthening of the programmes. Assistance was also provided to countries for developing their medium-term plans as well as annual work plans for the prevention and control of AIDS.

To mobilise national and inter-country efforts, WHO plays a very important advocacy role by highlighting the extent and potential impact of this pandemic on Asia as well as by emphasising the need to act now! The Regional Office produced and distributed a booklet called "AIDS in South-East Asia : No time for complacency", a video entitled "Facing the Challenge: AIDS in South-East Asia" and advocacy materials on school AIDS education including a video film, a story book and games. Various sectors are now being involved in AIDS prevention and control including NGOs and private sector in many countries. In January 1995, the Regional Office organised an inter-country meeting to enhance the involvement of private sector in HIV/AIDS prevention and in 1996 prepared a book "NGOs and AIDS: Responding to an expanding epidemic" to assist and guide NGOs in their work.

More recently, the Regional Office has provided technical and material support to ASEAN in development of their regional work programme, to Chulalongkorn University, Thailand, in a consultation on information on population movement and HIV/AIDS, to All India Institute of Medical Sciences to organise an international meeting on AIDS and Hepatitis and to Indian Law Institute in hosting an international Conference on HIV and Law.

In view of the association between HIV and STD and the role played by STD, particularly genital ulcer disease, in the acquisition and transmission of HIV, the Regional Office is promoting the need to strengthen STD services in the countries. Early diagnosis and treatment of STDs is being given a high priority as primary prevention measures against HIV infection. STD control is an important agenda item at annual meetings of programme managers. As a result, all the national programmes are now focusing their efforts on diagnosis of STD using syndromic approach and providing the most effective drugs at the first contact with health services. The STD management guidelines and training package has also been developed to assist countries.

A network for monitoring gonococcal antimicrobial susceptibility has also been established in the region. Priority is being assigned also to ensuring safe blood transfusions and blood products. To assist countries in this priority area, the Regional Office has developed a book entitled "Strategies for Safe Blood Transfusion" which has been widely distributed to member countries.

Indeed, experiences from countries both on prevention and care must be shared. With this in mind, the Regional Office convenes every year a meeting of the National AIDS Programme Managers. In November 1996, the Regional Office, in collaboration with and support from UNAIDS, invited all the AIDS programme managers to Dhaka to share their experiences in AIDS prevention and care. A quarterly newsletter AIDSWATCH is being published since October 1996 which is now accessible worldwide on internet.

In South-East Asia, patients with AIDS are increasingly being diagnosed and HIV/AIDS care is now becoming a major issue to be addressed in the region. To respond to this need, the Regional Office is promoting the concept of HIV/AIDS continuum of care at various levels i.e. institution, community and home. The concept proposes that HIV/AIDS care should be integrated with primary health care and that care at all levels should be strengthened in view of the anticipated increase in AIDS cases in the future. An inter-country meeting on the continuum of care was held in Bangkok in 1993 which provided a basis for planning care approaches in the Region.

The Regional Office has developed a number of technical documents on this subject including "HIV/AIDS Counselling: A module for trainers", "Understanding and Living with AIDS", and "HIV testing Policies and Strategies". These have been distributed for use by health care workers, NGOs as well as training institutions. The HQ home-care handbook has been adapted and distributed in Member Countries. Guidelines on "Prevention of HIV, HBV and other infections at health care settings" has also been prepared.

The AIDS has already emerged as a serious public health and developmental problem in the region. All the countries are concerned and have expressed their commitment to combat this expanding pandemic. The problem has been discussed in various fora, including the Meeting of Health Ministers, by other high-level government officials as well as NGOs and private sector. The situation is dynamic requiring continuous updating and sharing of information.

The World Bank's support to the South Asia region began with India in 1992. Since then, the strategy continues to emphasise prevention, health promotion in high risk populations, and the mitigation of high risk situations. World Bank assistance to South Asia, including planned commitments, totals over US$350 million equivalent. This support is closely coordinated with UN agencies and bilaterals.

Preventing AIDS epidemic is at the top of the agenda in South Asia. To void South Asia's hard-earned economic and social achievements is a global threat. In all nations of South Asia, preventing the AIDS epidemic and mitigating its impact must be at the centre of development policies and programmes.

REFERENCES

WHO's Report on HIV/AIDS in Asia and the Pacific region, 2001.

Sentinel Surveillance Data Resources, Department of Health, Myanmar, March, 1988.

UNAIDS Report on the Global HIV/AIDS Epidemic, 2002.

3

Combating HIV/AIDS in India

In India, the initial cases of HIV/AIDS were reported among commercial sex workers in Mumbai and Chennai and injecting drug users in the northeastern State of Manipur. The disease spread rapidly in the areas adjoining these epicentres and by 1996 Maharashtra, Tamil Nadu and Manipur together accounted for 77 per cent of the total AIDS cases with Maharashtra reporting almost half the number of cases in the country. Even though the officially reported cases of HIV infections and full-blown AIDS cases are in thousands only, it is realized that there is a wide gap between the reported and estimated figures because of the absence of epidemiological data in major parts of the country. The overall prevalence in the country for a population of 970 million is still however, very low, a rate much lower than many other countries in the Asia-Pacific region.

Within a short period AIDS has emerged as one of the most serious public health problem in the country. In the recent years it has spread from urban to rural areas and from individuals practising risk behaviour to the general population. Studies indicate that more and more women attending anti-natal clinics are testing HIV-positive thereby increasing the risk of prenatal transmission. About 75 per cent of the infections occur from the sexual route (both heterosexual and homosexual), about 8 per cent through blood transfusion, another 8 per cent through injecting drug use. About 89 per cent of the reported cases are occurring in sexually active and economically productive age group of 18-40 years. One in every 4 cases reported is a woman. The attributable factors for such rapid spread of the epidemic across the country today is labour migration and mobility in search of employment from economically backward to more advanced regions, low literacy levels leading to low awareness among the potential high risk groups, gender disparity, Sexually Transmitted Infections and Reproductive Tract Infections both among men and women.

The social stigma attached to sexually transmitted infections also hold good for HIV / AIDS, even in a much more serious manner. This, coupled with lack of awareness, results in reporting of full-blown AIDS cases in cities like Mumbai and Chennai causing severe strain on the hospital infrastructure. There have been cases of refusal of AIDS patients in hospitals and nursing homes both in Government and private sectors. This has compounded the misery of the AIDS patients. More often it is mistaken to be a contagious disease and patients are isolated in the wards creating a scare among the general patients. In the workplace there were cases of discrimination leading, in some occasions, to loss of employment.

The active part played by some non-Governmental organisations in bringing out public interest litigations against such cases of discrimination and the judicial pronouncements by courts in support of the rights of such people has helped in alleviating the misery of the affected persons. The treatment options are still in the initial trial stage and are prohibitively expensive. While there is no vaccine in sight at least till now, multi-drug protease inhibitor therapy, popularly known as 'cocktail therapy', is not a cure to the disease and may help only in prolonging the life of the patient. Therapeutic trials of these drugs are still in an elementary stage and there are fears of patients developing drug resistance and side effects if the therapy is not administered under proper medical supervision. There were instances of quacks taking advantage of the situation and promising cure through so-called herbal treatment and defrauding unsuspecting people who are infected with the virus of large sums of money.

Transmission of the disease through blood, though issue as unsuspecting population can get infected through this route if safe blood is not ensured. Existence of a large number of small and medium blood banks, many of them in the private sector, also compounds the problem. The Supreme Court directive of May, 1996 has helped in phasing out unlicensed blood banks by May, 1997 and the prospective phasing out of professional blood donors by December, 1997. Compulsory testing of blood for HIV along with Syphilis, Malaria and Hepatitis B, which has now been introduced throughout the country will help in checking transmission of HIV virus through blood transfusion.

The problem of injecting drug users is not universal and is restricted to the northeastern States and the urban pockets of metropolitan cities. The injecting needles which are the principal cause of transmission in such cases are used repeatedly by the drug users. The twin problem of drug addiction and HIV transmission pose a serious ethical and moral problem in the HIV prevention programme. Needle exchange programmes which have been taken up in other countries to ensure availability of sterile needles for drug users are frowned upon in India because of ethical and moral implications.

Although transmission of HIV through use of needles, razors and other cutting instruments in the thousands of beauty parlours, hair-cutting saloons and dental is insignificant, lack of hygienic practices in majority of these establishments also poses a health risk to the unsuspecting general population who visit these places every day. There is a great necessity in bringing these establishments to acceptable standards of hygiene to minimise and almost eliminate the chances of HIV transmission through the use of needles and sharp cutting instruments.

With about 14 million TB cases existing in India, HIV/AIDS also poses a twin challenge of HIV/TB co-infection. Nearly 60 per cent of the AIDS cases are reported to be opportunistic TB infection cases. Treatment of TB among the HIV-infected persons is a new challenge to the National TB Control Programme which has now adopted DOTS strategy for control of TB infection. Some of the drugs which are recommended for TB treatment pose complications in cases of HIV-infected persons and had to be withdrawn in areas of high HIV prevalence. At the same time looking for HIV among TB infected persons will also cause the problem of scaring away of a large number of TB infected cases in the country from seeking treatment under the DOTS strategy. There is no risk of any TB patient getting infected with HIV unless he or she practises high risk behaviour or gets infected from transfusion of HIV-infected blood.

HIV/AIDS is not a disease which spreads randomly and is transmitted as a consequence of a specific behavioural pattern and has strong socioeconomic implications. It not only costs huge sums of money in terms of controlling the opportunistic infections such as TB, Pneumonia and cryptococcal meningitis, but seriously affects individuals in their prime productive years causing serious economic loss to them and their families.

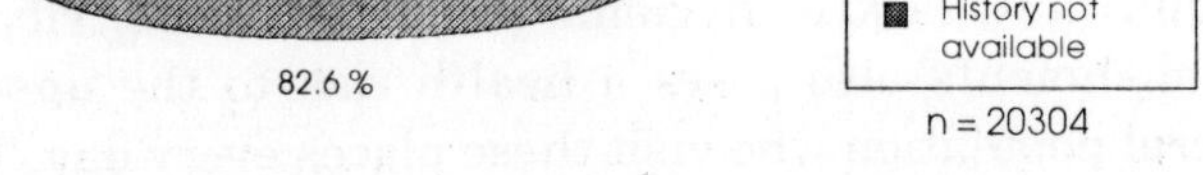

Figure 1: Probable sources of infections in AIDS cases in India, May 1986-March 2001

In India with a large population and population density, low literacy levels and consequent low levels of awareness, HIV/AIDS is one of the most challenging health problems ever faced by the country. Soon after reporting of the first HIV/AIDS case in the country, the Government recognised the seriousness of the problem and took a series of important measures to tackle the epidemic.

A high-powered National AIDS Committee was constituted in 1986 itself and a National AIDS Control Programme was launched a year later. In the initial years the programme focused on generation of public awareness through mass communication programmes, introduction of blood screening for transfusion purposes and conducting surveillance activities in the epicentres of the epidemic. In 1992 the Government formulated a multi-sectoral strategy for the prevention and control of AIDS in India. It is implemented through the National AIDS Control Organisation at the national level and State AIDS Cells/Societies at the State/UT levels.

Several important actions have been taken to ensure safe blood by modernisation and strengthening of blood banks, introduction of licensing system of blood banks and gradual phasing out of professional blood donors. Introduction of component separation facilities has also helped in reducing the use of whole blood for transfusion. Some very successful intervention programmes among the high risk groups like commercial sex workers in the Sonagachi area of Calcutta, men having sex with men in Chennai and injecting drug users in Manipur were carried out through the dedicated involvement of non-Governmental organisations. Availability of good quality condoms through social marketing has made a significant increase in the last three years.

The inexorable spread of the disease from the initial epicentre to the rest of the country underscores the immediate need to have a paradigm shift in the response against HIV/AIDS at all levels making it imperative to formulate a comprehensive national policy on HIV/AIDS in order to cope effectively with the changed nature of the HIV/AIDS problem. The entire programme of prevention and control of HIV/AIDS needs a shift towards a more holistic approach looking at AIDS as a developmental problem instead of a mere public health issue. For this purpose a series of deliberations have been held with representatives of doctors, scientists, social workers, NGOs and other eminent personalities working in the field of HIV/AIDS prevention and control. Technical Working Groups constituted to address various aspects of HIV/AIDS prevention and control strategy have given valuable output.

ESTIMATES OF HIV/AIDS (HIV SENTINEL SURVEILLANCE ROUND-2000)

As the Sentinel surveillance system has been established as the best system to monitor trends of HIV infection in specific high risk groups as well as low risk groups, it was decided to adopt Sentinel surveillance methodology. Few selected sentinel sites representing the various groups of population would be screened for HIV prevalence and its trends are monitored over a period of time. Accordingly the Sentinel surveillance for HIV infection was taken up in 55 sentinel sites in 1994, which was expanded, to 180 Sentinel Sites in 1998 in various parts of the country. The population groups and sites are chosen based on information of risk behaviour of various risk groups for HIV infection. The high-risk groups of population include patients attending Sexually Transmitted Diseases (STD), clinics and intravenous drug users while low risk of population includes mothers attending antenatal clinics. The rationale of choosing Sentinel sites in these clinics, is that the samples from people with risk behaviour of multi-partner sex and IVDUs attending these clinic based settings will be collected on regular intervals. The whole procedure is "Unlinked Anonymous".

Every year from August to October, a round of survey is conducted in the designated sites. During year 2000, the survey was conducted in 232 sites with inclusion of 57 new sites and deletion of 5 sites from the existing list. These sites include 109 sites in STD clinics, 110 sites in Antenatal clinics, 11 sites among IDUs and 2 sites for MSM. The data thus collected, was analysed by NIHFW to assess trends of HIV prevalence rates among identified risk groups over the years. 45 districts mostly in high prevalent States have shown high prevalence of HIV among STD & ANC during this round. A statement indicating State-wise locations of districts with high HIV prevalence is enclosed.

The HIV prevalence in adult population can be broadly classified into three groups of States/UTs in the country.

Group I: States like Maharasthra, Tamil Nadu, Karnataka, Andhra Pradesh, Manipur and Nagaland where the HIV infection has crossed 1 per cent or more in antenatal women.

Group II: States like Gujrat, Goa and Pondicherry where HIV infection has crossed 5 per cent or more among high risk groups but the infection is below 1 per cent in antenatal women.

Group III: Remaining States where the HIV infection in any of the high risk groups is still less than 5 per cent and is less than 1 per cent among antenatal women.

It can be inferred from the Sentinel surveillance data from antenatal clinics in 7 metro cities in the country, that HIV infection has crossed 2 per cent in Mumbai, is more than 1 per cent in Hyderabad. Bangalore, Chennai and is below 1 per cent in Calcutta, Ahmedabad and Delhi. This data clearly supports the evidence that HIV infection is percolating from various high risk groups to general population.

Estimation of HIV Infection among Adult Population

In the Indian context, it is difficult to estimate the exact prevalence of HIV because of the varied cultural characteristics, traditions and values with special reference to sex related risk behaviours. The western African model of making estimates cannot be easily applied to the Indian scenario. However, it is possible to have rough estimates with range, that may be used for planning of AIDS Prevention and

Control Programme. These estimates can also be useful for mapping of specific vulnerable groups and areas to plan targeted interventions in major urban and other areas in the States. To estimate the total burden of HIV infections in the country, some efforts had been made in the past by World Health Organisation (WHO/UNAIDS), by using the data generated by NACO and other publications from various Research Institutes in India. Although the HIV sentinel surveillance data has been primarily used for monitoring the trends i.e. to assess how rapidly HIV infection increases or decreases over time in different groups and areas, it can also provide an estimate of the total burden of HIV infection in the country.

The Sentinel surveillance programme was expanded in 1998, to cover 180 sentinel sites in the country. During year 2000, we had established 57 additional sites and this round was conducted in 232 sites. The data thus generated had certain strengths like consistency, availability of data from rural sentinel sites and representativeness from various risk groups. This has provided an opportunity to work out the total burden of HIV infection in the country.

The concept of using HIV sentinel data to estimate the burden of HIV infection was brought out in the WHO document "HIV/AIDS/STD Surveillance Data—Management and Use" of August 1996. The document suggests that sero surveys of Sentinel population is often the most popular method of estimating the burden of HIV infection. A reliable estimate can be made by using data from sero prevalence studies of different sub populations at different levels of risk and the HIV prevalence level is applied to the population which the study group represents. For example, in epidemics where heterosexual transmission is predominant, the HIV prevalence rate in antenatal women is applied to sexually active population (15 – 49 years). For estimating HIV prevalence among various risk groups, an estimation of the size of these groups is necessary. The caution here is that risk groups should not overlap.

Such estimates are made by applying the following formula:

$$V = (P/T)(R)$$

Here V is the total estimate, P is the number of HIV positive, T is the number of samples tested and R is the estimated size of population.

As the extent of reliability of HIV estimate will depend upon the accuracy of the estimation of size of risk group population, careful assumptions are required in respect of various parameters like urban rural mix, male female ratio, STD prevalence in urban and rural areas etc. Various assumptions were evolved after intensive interaction with noted epidemiologists and Bio-statisticians in the country through a process of consultation. The following assumptions on different parameters for estimation of the size of the risk group populations have been recommended.

i) The 1991 census figures and the projected figures for 2000 will be the basis for State specific assumptions for:
   a) Midyear population (in the age group of 15-49 years)
   b) Urban population and rural population
   c) Male-Female ratio

ii) STD prevalence rates in both urban and rural populations as follows:
   a) STD prevalence in urban areas will be 10 per cent in high prevalent States, 7 per cent in medium prevalent States and 5 per cent in low prevalent States. It will be the same for both males and females.
   b) 5 per cent prevalence in rural populations in all States/UTs, for both males and females.

iii) For the purpose of HIV estimation in high-risk population, urban rural differential will be 3:1 in all the States. Similarly, for HIV prevalence in low risk population, the urban-rural differential will be 8:1 in all the States.

vi) As there are more infected males than females, the following ratio would be applied:

In high prevalent States, for every infected female there are 1.2 males, in moderate prevalent States, for every infected female there are 2 males and in low prevalence States, for every infected female there will be 3 males.

Similarly, for every male STD patient from highly prevalent States, it is assumed that there would be 0.83 females, for moderate prevalent States, there will be 0.5 females and for low prevalent States, there would be 0.33 female patients.

v) In respect of the HIV prevalence rates:

The median value of HIV prevalence from State specific and group specific Sentinel data has been applied:

For States where the HIV prevalence rate has been reported as "0", the following assumptions are made.

a) If data were available from previous round where the prevalence is more than '0', the rate from the previous round will be adopted.

b) If the previous round data also shows '0' prevalence the arithmetic mean of the low prevalent States will be applicable in place of "0" value.

vi) For estimation of HIV infection among IVDUs, the HIV prevalence rate will be applied to the estimated size of IVDUs population in the State.

vii) The States will be categorised as high, moderate or low, based on following definition:

High prevalent States: States where HIV prevalence in antenatal women is 1 per cent or more.

Moderate prevalent states: States where the HIV prevalence in antenatal women is less than 1 per cent and prevalence in STD and other high risk groups is 5 per cent or more.

Low prevalent states: States where the HIV prevalence in antenatal women is less than 1 per cent and HIV prevalence among STD and other high-risk group is less than 5 per cent.

Based on these assumptions a worksheet was developed to estimate the number of HIV infection in adult population in the country. This data was examined by small working group of Epidemiologists and Bio-statisticians at NIHFW. Finally, the data was presented to "Task Force on Surveillance" for discussion and finalisation of output. Using these assumptions and consistence methodology, estimates of HIV infections have been worked out during 1998, 1999 and this year i.e. 2000. A range of 20 per cent is applied to the point estimate, to provide higher and lower values on this estimate. Keeping in view, the fact that all risk groups are not adequately represented, age groups excluding 15-49 years are not included and AIDS cases are not included in this exercise, upper side of the range has been taken as working estimate for the country, as per details given below:

1998	3.50 million
1999	3.70 million
2000	3.86 million

The justification for urban-rural and male-female gradient is as follows:

i) It is assumed that HIV spreads from urban to rural area and this differential is maintained even at very high level of HIV prevalence.

ii) It is assumed that higher percentage of males have risk behaviour as compared to females in India. In the beginning of the epidemic, males outnumber females and ratio gets closer to 1 with the progression of the epidemic in general population. In all the South Asian countries, males outnumber females.

iii) It is also assumed that the infection shifts from high-risk population to general population over a period of time. Therefore, all the States go through a stage of low and then concentrated and finally generalised epidemic in the absence of effective interventions.

NATIONAL AIDS CONTROL PROGRAMME I (1999-2004)

The National AIDS Control Programme has become effective from 9th November, 1999. It is a 100 per cent Centrally sponsored scheme implemented in 32 States/UTs and three Municipal Corporations namely Ahmedabad, Chennai and Mumbai through AIDS Control Societies. The three new states of Chattisgarh, Uttaranchal and Jharkhand are in the process of establishing their State AIDS Control Societies.

The National AIDS Control Project has two key objectives

i) to reduce the spread of HIV infection in India;
ii) to strengthen India's capacity to respond to HIV/AIDS on a long term basis.

Operationally, the project interventions would seek to achieve the following by the end of the project:

i) to keep HIV prevalence rate below 5 per cent of adult population in Maharashtra, below 3 per cent in Andhra Pradesh, Karnataka, Manipur, Tamil Nadu where the HIV prevalence is moderate and below 1 per cent in remaining States, where the epidemic is still at a nascent stage;
ii) to reduce blood borne transmission of HIV to less than 1 per cent
iii) to attain awareness level of not less than 90 per cent among the youth and others in the reproductive age group; and
iv) to achieve condom use of not less than 90 per cent among high risk categories like Commercial Sex Workers.

The programme has the following firm targets to be achieved during project period:

i) To reduce blood-borne transmission of HIV to less than one per cent of the total transmissions.

ii) To introduce Hepatitis C as the fifth mandatory test for blood screening.

iii) To set up 10 new modern blood banks in uncovered areas, upgrading of 20 major blood banks, setting up of 80 new district level blood banks in uncovered districts, establishing another 40 blood component separation units, promotion of voluntary blood donation and increase its share in total blood collected to at least 60 per cent. The total blood collection in the county which is now around 3-3.5 million units is sought to be raised to 5-5.5 million units by the end of the project.

iv) To attain awareness level of not less than 90 per cent among the youth and those in the reproductive age group.

v) To train up at least 600 NGOs in the country in conducting targeted intervention programmes among high-risk groups and through them promote condom use of not less than 90 per cent among these groups and control of STDs.

vi) To conduct annual Family Health Awareness Campaigns among the general population and provide service-delivery in terms of medical advice and provision of drugs for control of STDs and Reproductive Tract Infections (RTIs). These campaigns will be conducted jointly by NACO and RHC programme managers at the State level.

vii) Promotion of voluntary testing facilities across the country at the end of the project. It is visualised that every district in the country would have at least one voluntary testing facility.

viii) Awareness campaigns will now be more interactive and use of traditional media such as folk arts and street theatre will be given greater priority in the rural areas. It is proposed to cover all the schools in the country targeting students studying in Class IX and Class XI through school education programmes and all the universities through the "Universities. Talk AIDS" programme during the project period.

ix) Promotion of Organisations of people living with HIV/AIDS and giving them financial support to form self-help groups.

Components of Phase II

i) *Priority targeted interventions for populations at high risk*: This component of the project aims to reduce the spread of HIV in groups at high risk by identifying target populations and providing peer counselling, condom promotion, treatment of sexually transmitted infections etc. This component is delivered largely through Non Government Organisations, Community based Organisations and the Public sector.

ii) *Preventive interventions for the general population*: The main activities are:

a) IEC and awareness campaigns;

b) provide voluntary testing and counselling;

c) reduction of transmission by blood transfusion; and

d) prevention of occupational exposure.

iii) *Low cost care for people living with HIV/AIDS*: Under this component financial and technical assistance is provided to States/UTs for home based and community based care, including increasing the availability of cost effective interventions for common opportunistic infections.

iv) *Institutional strengthening:* This component aims to strengthen effectiveness and technical managerial and financial sustainability at National, State and Municipal levels; strengthening surveillance activities and building strong Research & Development component, including operational research etc.

v) *Inter-sectoral collaboration:* This component promotes collaboration amongst the public, private and voluntary sectors. The activities would be coordinated with other programmes within the Ministry of Health & Family Welfare and other central ministries and departments. Collaboration would focused on;

vi) Learning from the innovative HIV/AIDS programmes that exist in other sectors; and

vii) Sharing in the working, generating awareness, advocacy and delivering interventions.

Outlay for National AIDS Control Programme- II

There are three funding agencies for Phase II of National AIDS Control Programme. These are :

i) *International Development Agency (IDA)*: World Bank has provided an account of US $191.00 million as soft loan for the project and the domestic budgetary support is US $ 38.8 million. The total outlay is US $ 229.8 million (Rs. 11550.00 million).

ii) *United States Agency for International Development (USAID)*: United States Agency for International Development has extended its assistance to the Govt. of Maharashtra for implementation of 'AVERT' Project based on their earlier experience of working in the State of Tamil Nadu under the AIDS Prevention and AIDS Control (APAC) project. The outlay for USAID assisted 'AVERT' project is Rs. 1660.00 million.

iii) *Department For International Development (DFID) of UK Government*: Department For International Development has extended its assistance for implementation of Sexual Health Projects in the States of Andhra Pradesh, Gujarat, Kerala and Orissa in continuation of their earlier projects in West Bengal. The outlay for this project is Rs. 1040.00 million.

Outlay for national AIDS control project phase - II	*Rupees in million*
IDA credit (1999-2004)	11550
USAID assistance for AVERT Project in Maharashtra.	1660
DFID assistance for Sexual Health projects for the States of Andhra Pradesh, Gujarat, Kerala and Orissa.	1040
Total	14250

For the effective monitoring and evaluation to assess the implementation of the Phase-II of the National AIDS Control Project at National and State level, the following mechanism has been envisaged.

i) Creating a Computerised Management Information System (CMIS) at the National and State levels;
ii) Training NACO Staff and Health specialists in evidence based health programme management.
iii) Conducting base line, mid term and final evaluation;
iv) Conducting the Annual Performance and Expenditure Review (APER); and
v) Conducting the National Performance Review (NPR) under the National AIDS Control Board.

Following are the major achievements of the national AIDS control programme:

i) National AIDS Prevention & Control Policy drafted to prevent the HIV infection from further spread and reduce the socioeconomic impact of HIV/AIDS.
ii) To ensure easily accessible and adequate supply of safe blood and blood product, the National Blood Policy drafted.

iii) All district Women's hospitals strengthened for management of Reproductive Tract Infections including Sexually Transmitted Diseases in addition to STD clinics functioning in Medical colleges and district hospitals.

iv) Voluntary Blood Testing Centres have been established in medical colleges and major hospitals to facilitate testing for HIV with pre-test and post-test counselling.

v) Districts are being covered in a phased manner in 2-3 years all over the country. Financial support provided to all States for management of "Opportunistic Infections" for people living with HIV/AIDS.

vi) Annual rounds of Sentinel Surveillance for HIV infection were carried out during August-October at various sites (Antenatal Clinics, STD Clinics and Intravenous Drug Users) to understand the nature and spread of epidemic and to study the trend.

vii) Hon'ble Prime Minister of India addressed Members of Parliament from Lok Sabha and Rajya Sabha to sensitise them to the problem of HIV/AIDS. Chief Ministers/ Health Ministers of six high prevalence States were also addressed by Hon'ble Prime Minister.

viii) Hon'ble Prime Minister convened a meeting of captains of business houses in India and appealed to them to form business coalition to deal with the problem of HIV/AIDS effectively at workplaces in collaboration with public and NGO sectors.

ix) Targetted Intervention projects for poor and marginalised high risk groups have been initiated by all States and UTs. These projects aimed at providing reproductive health care services, Promotion of condom use and counselling.

x) Specific guidelines have been developed to encourage participation of Non-Government Organisations (NGOs) in HIV/AIDS Prevention and Control Programme.

xi) For the expeditious flow of funds and implementation of the programmes, State AIDS Control Societies have been constituted in all States/UTs with adequate technical and managerial staff.

xii) Community care centres have been established in States with high prevalence of HIV.

xiii) For the protection of medical and para-medical workers attending HIV/AIDS cases, from acquiring HIV infection in case they get accidental injury like needle prick/sharp injury, provision has been made to provide post exposure prophylaxis using anti-retroviral drugs.

xiv) Collaboration with Ministries/Deptt. of Defence, Railways, Sports and Youth Affairs, Employees' State Insurance Corporation and Steel Authority of India, Social Justice and Empowerment etc., in HIV/AIDS prevention and control programme.

xv) Initiation of School AIDS Education Programme by all States/UTs involvement of Deptt. of Education and NGOs.

xvi) Conduction of National Family Health Awareness Campaign twice a year to sensitise community, particularly in urban slums and rural area about Sexually Transmitted Diseases and HIV/AIDS. The last round of the campaign was held during the period April-June, 2001.

xvii) A comprehensive training programme for Medical and Para-medical workers have been initiated to train them in prevention and control of HIV/AIDS.

xviii) A feasibility study of prevention of Mother to Child Transmission of HIV by administering short course AZT is under implementation in 11 centres in States of Maharashtra, Tamil Nadu, Karnataka, Andhra Pradesh and Manipur.

PREVENTION OF HIV/AIDS

The Prime Minister of India met the Chief Ministers of the six high prevalence states of Andhra Pradesh, Karnataka, Maharashtra, Tamil Nadu, Manipur and Nagaland on May 22, 2001 to intensify implementation of comprehensive strategic in prevention and control of HIV/AIDS in their states. He stated political advocacy and commitment at national and state levels is critical for effective implementation of National AIDS Control Programme. Govt. of India has consistently shown highest level of commitment towards control of HIV/AIDS infection since inception of the National Programme.

The Union Health Minister also highlighted the importance of sensitive leadership and supervision from highest political level in intensifying the efforts for checking the spread of HIV/AIDS. The Chief Ministers responded positively to the initiatives taken by the Prime Minister and assured him that they would keep HIV/AIDS on top priority in view of the high prevalence of the infection in their respective States. They accorded primacy to school and college based educational programmes, involvement of informal leaders in spreading the message of HIV/AIDS and enlisting the support of community leaders. The Chief Ministers requested the Government of India to increase funding for priority areas of the programme like support to hospital infection control measures, provision of medicines for opportunistic infections and prevention of mother-to-child transmission. The Prime Minister also highlighted the importance of involving religious leaders for dissemination information about HIV/AIDS prevention and control among the people.

The UN General Assembly's Special session on HIV/AIDS (UNGASS) was held in New York between 25th and 27th June 2001. In this session, a "Declaration of Commitment" was adopted laying emphasis on the Prevention and Control of HIV/AIDS and Care of people living with AIDS. The delegates agreed to establish a Global HIV/AIDS and Health Fund to combat this epidemic. The Indian delegation at the UN Special session was lead by Union Minister of Health. Smt. Sonia Gandhi, Leader of Opposition and MP in the Parliament, in her address to the august gathering assured India's deep commitment at the highest political level to do everything possible to control this epidemic.

The Prime Minister met business leaders and industrialists on 1st December 2000 to develop a Government-Business partnership to control the further spread of HIV / AIDS in the country. The Business Leaders assured the Prime Minister that they will form a Business Coalition Trust for HIV/AIDS to coordinate and fund AIDS control efforts in organised and unorganised sectors of industry.

The Blood Safety Programme of NACO assists in ensuring the adequacy and safety of blood supply in the country. The National and State Blood Transfusion Councils, funded mainly by NACO, are also supplementing Blood Safety activity in the States. The National Blood Policy has been formulated for better management and assurance of blood and blood products and is expected to act as a policy framework for further activities.

The State AIDS Control Societies are encouraged to develop IEC materials and plan programmes for promoting voluntary non remunerated blood donation which has shown some increase in the recent past. Some of the states like Maharashtra and West Bengal have made considerable progress in this area.

Besides raising awareness, in general, regarding safety of blood and blood products, NACO is also encouraging training of all Blood Transfusion Services staff by providing financial assistance in the annual action plan of States.

From 1st June, 2001, it is made mandatory to test all donated blood for Hepatitis C Virus antibodies, besides testing for Hepatitis B, HIV, Syphilis and Malaria which are already implemented. With the help of National Institute of Biologicals, an EQAS programme is being instituted wherein it is planned to involve blood bank laboratories also.

In order to improve standards for good manufacturing practices in blood banks, a major thrust is put on Quality Management Training programmes. Workshops for training of blood bank personnel and sensitisation of programme officers of states are conducted with the help of WHO to ensure application of quality systems.

In order to ease the situation of shortages in the rural areas and in smaller hospitals where it is not feasible to operate blood banks, it is now planned to establish storage centres which can provide tested blood obtained from district blood banks for life threatening emergencies.

In the underserved states, state-of-the-art blood centres are being developed. These centres will be provided equipment and it is proposed that NACO would manage such centres for a period of time before handing them over to the State Governments. It is expected that during this period staff will be fully trained to implement quality systems and gain confidence of all users. These centres will also be networked with the existing blood banks in the areas to improve optimal use of available blood.

The Technical Resource Group of Blood Safety meets regularly and is shortly producing a manual on "Best Practices in BTS". For appropriate use of blood, recent WHO publications on the subject are being widely distributed especially in Medical Colleges to make the students and clinical users of blood aware of the importance of this field.

IEC STRATEGY

Communication continues to be one of the most important strategies in the fight against HIV/AIDS. In the absence of a vaccine or a cure, prevention is the most effective strategy for the control of HIV/AIDS. In India, the majority of the population is still uninfected. It, therefore, becomes imperative to continue intensive communication efforts that will not only raise awareness levels but also bring out behaviour change. Information, Education and Communication (IEC) is a process that informs, motivates and helps people to adopt and maintain healthy practices and life skills. It aims at empowering individuals and enabling them to make correct decisions about safe behaviour practices. IEC also attempts to create an environment, which is conducive, and supports access to treatment and services for those already infected. If communication has to be effective it must be in the local language, keeping in mind social norms, cultural beliefs and sensitivities of the community.

All communication programmes must give space for interaction, clarifying doubts, addressing misgivings on the issues of sex and sexuality, which are traditionally not discussed openly in a conservative society. In India, therefore, development of appropriate and effective IEC strategies for HIV/AIDS is one of the biggest challenges not only in the health but also in the development sector. In the NACP-II, NACO is giving the highest priority to an effective and sustained strategy to bring about changes in behaviour to prevent further infection. For an effective IEC campaign, a full range of activities and approaches—from mass media campaigns for public education to the use of targeted interventions to help individuals negotiate safer practices—is being used. IEC programmes have also been integrated in various components of the programme such as STD services, Condom promotion and Blood safety.

Many studies have been conducted to ascertain the knowledge, attitude, behaviour and practices of the people in general as well as those who practice high risk behaviour in the context of AIDS and STDs. These studies had limited target groups, but provide baseline information for developing programme strategies. Certain common findings emerge from the studies. These are:

i) Most individuals do not have accurate and complete information on HIV/AIDS.

ii) The link between STD and AIDS is not clear to most people.

iii) STDs are not taken seriously, since they are curable.

iv) There is a belief that HIV transmission and AIDS is found in only limited groups, such as foreigners, homosexuals, sex workers and drug users.

v) The IEC campaign and targeted interventions have demonstrated changes in knowledge, perception and behaviour.

vi) A Prevention Indicator Study has demonstrated a rise in awareness levels from 68 per cent to 94 per cent in some of the urban areas and 9 per cent to 35 per cent in rural areas.

The IEC strategy in NACO is operationalised at two levels. At the national level, it focuses on political and media advocacy. At field level it addresses issues such as creation of a supportive environment that reduces social stigma and discrimination and promotion of utilisation of services. NACO has set up an IEC division at headquarters comprising of a Joint Director, Deputy Director, Under Secretary and National Consultants. This division is responsible for developing the IEC policy, strategy, and guidelines both at the national and state level. It is also responsible for monitoring and supervising the IEC activities undertaken by the State AIDS Control Societies.

At the state level the IEC activities have been decentralised keeping in mind the need to respond to local priorities and to facilitate communication in local languages. In order to create baseline data for the AIDS-II Project, NACO has directed the State AIDS Control Societies to conduct a Communication Needs Assessment in every state on the basis of which a state level IEC plan will be developed. NACO has also formulated IEC guidelines to provide a framework for focused and cost effective IEC activities. The objectives of the IEC strategy in the National AIDS Control Programme are:

i) To raise awareness, improve knowledge and understanding among the general population about AIDS infection and STD, routes of transmission and method of prevention.

ii) To promote desirable practices such as avoiding multi partner sex, condom use, sterilisation of needles/syringes and voluntary donation of blood.

iii) To mobilise all sectors of society to integrate messages and programmes on AIDS into their existing activities.

iv) To train health workers in AIDS communication and coping strategies for strengthening technical and managerial capabilities.

v) To create a supportive environment for the care and rehabilitation of persons with HIV/AIDS.

The IEC strategic plan for AIDS prevention and control programme in India includes, a variety of communication strategies for raising awareness, behavioural change and social mobilisation. The IEC strategic plan has the following components:

i) Use of mass media

ii) Advocacy at various levels

iii) Inter-sectoral collaboration

iv) Training

v) Involvement of NGOs

vi) Research.

National Level IEC Activities

NACO has empanelled two professional agencies to design and develop mass media campaigns on HIV/AIDS prevention and control in the country. These two agencies were selected through a transparent and competitive process and recommended by a committee of experts. In addition, NACO is utilising the various media units of the Ministry of Information and Broadcasting such as Directorate of Advertising and Visual Publicity, Directorate of Field Publicity, Song and Drama Division and the Press Information Bureau for out-reach in the rural areas and the regional press.

Electronic Media

NACO is utilising the massive out-reach of Doordarshan and private satellite channel for telecast of messages on HIV/AIDS prevention and control during prime time. These include messages on sexually transmitted diseases, blood safety and voluntary blood donation. Some of the specific activities are as follows:

i) *Spirit of unity concert:* NACO has sponsored a classical music programme "Spirit of Unity Concerts" to mainstream the issue of HIV/AIDS and to reach out to the cultural elite and other educated classes through this programme.

ii) *All India Radio:* A special programme, in the drama mode, has been devised for rural and migrant youth. The programme which is titled "Jiyo Aur Jeene Do" is being broadcast on 30 commercial broadcasting stations of AIR since June, 1998. The ten minutes programme is broadcast in 12 languages on Tuesday evening at 8.00 P.M.

iii) *AIR-FM:* NACO is using the popular FM channel to combine entertainment and education in reaching out to the urban youth. The one-hour programme which is titled "NACO Film Hit Parade" is broadcast for one hour every week on the AIR-FM channel in Delhi. The programme has received a wide and positive response from a number of people who respond on the telephone numbers given seeking medical advice and counselling.

iv) *Campaign for youth:* NACO developed two audio and two video spots focusing on the vulnerability of young people to HIV. The video spots were prepared in an animation format and were telecast on Doordarshan and satellite channels. The two radio spots were broadcast extensively on All India Radio. Press advertisements were also developed as part of this campaign. It is now proposed to evaluate the impact of this campaign before undertaking new activities.

v) *Voluntary blood donation:* Voluntary Blood Donation Day was observed on October 1, 2000. Various activities to mobilise voluntary blood donation was carried out throughout the country. Press advertisements were released in leading national dailies.

vi) *World AIDS day 2000:* The World AIDS Day was observed throughout the country on December 1, 2000. At the national level various activities were undertaken.

The Prime Minister met business leaders and industrialists on 1st December 2000 to develop a Government-Business partnership to control the further spread of HIV/AIDS in the country. The meeting was attended by the Union Health Minister, leading industrialists from various parts of the country, senior officials from the Prime Minister's Office, Ministries of Health & Family Welfare, Commerce, Railways Planning commission and business associations like CII, FICCI and ASSOCHAM. The meeting was also attended by representatives from UNAIDS, USAID, World Bank and DFID.

In continuation of the activities for the World AIDS Day, NACO in collaboration with UNICEF organised a panel discussion. Ms. Jaya Prada, Member of Parliament- Rajya Sabha inaugurated the panel discussion. The panel discussions included voices of young people their vulnerabilities and capabilities, the national perspective, young people as activists not victims, vulnerabilities and capabilities of HIV positive people and rights perspective with respect to young people. The panel discussion was followed by a play titled "The BIG A", produced by Spot Light production. The duration of the play was two hours. It takes an honest, heart warming and humorous look at HIV/AIDS – the patients, their families and the society around them. Full of music, movement and comedy, interspersed with depth and poignancy, the play entertains, while it engages your mind and heart.

Advocacy campaigns at all levels in civil society have been initiated to provide a momentum to the control and prevention efforts and to integrate the issue of HIV/AIDS in a wider multi-sectoral response.

Political leaders: Activities with political leaders and other elected people's representatives have been initiated to build support for the National Programme.

Religious leaders: Activities with religious leaders to create an enabling and positive environment are being taken up.

Industry and other sectors: The role of the business sector is important because a widespread epidemic can have serious repercussions on the economic development of the country. Activities with business leaders and other partner ministries for workplace interventions have been initiated. Opinion leaders in civil society are being sensitised on the issue.

Since 1994, the Song and Drama Division of Government of India has been involved in the AIDS awareness campaign. It has produced several street plays, songs and dramas and has performed in 400 different locations utilising the local drama troupes in many States. The Directorate of Field Publicity has also participated in the campaign. All its 260 units located countrywide have conducted several programmes such as seminars, debate/essay and quiz competitions and film shows for AIDS awareness. An increasing number of programmes are also being carried out through various radio stations in the country by arranging panel discussions, features, phone-in programmes etc. The Press Information Bureau of the Government of India has organised a number of programmes to sensitise the regional press on the issue of HIV/AIDS.

National AIDS Telephone Helpline

A toll free National AIDS Telephone Helpline has been set up to provide access to information and counselling on HIV/AIDS related issues. This is a computerised four-digit number, 1097, with a voice response system linked with the telephonic hotline. This is a very popular service, since it maintains the confidentiality of the callers and helps the caller clarify doubts and access personal counselling without revealing their identity. The helpline number 1097 has become a very popular service in 77 cities and towns all over the country.

School AIDS Education Programme

Young people are among the most vulnerable to HIV/AIDS. School AIDS Education is one of the important programmes that focuses towards student youth to raise awareness levels, help young people resist peer pressure and develop a safe and responsible lifestyle. The programme reinforces family values and respect for the opposite sex. The activities include training of teachers and peer educators among students, role-playing, debates and discussions, question box and access to referral services, if necessary. Many States have already initiated programmes under this scheme. To bring about uniformity in approach, a training module called" Learning For Life" has been prepared and distributed to all states.

University Talk AIDS (UTA) Project

The University Talk AIDS (UTA) Project began in October 1991 and is a collaborative partnership between the National Service Scheme (NSS), Dept. of Youth Affairs & Sports and NACO. The project involves creating awareness among students and the youth on issues related to HIV/AIDS through workshops, seminars and written materials especially designed for them. Evaluation of the project has indicated that it has reached 7595 institutions and 6.5 million youth all across the country. The

UTA initiative employs an interactive and participatory approach that involves youth in finding relevant solutions themselves to the prevention of HIV/AIDS spread through their high –risk behaviour and lifestyle. It has been successful in creating awareness on HIV/AIDS and has developed responsible attitudes towards sex among the student youth. The information deals not only with HIV/AIDS but also with other important issues for the youth such as drug abuse, relationships, courtship and marriage etc. The key message is to delay the first sexual experience and adopt safe sex practices.

Nehru Yuvak Kendras

The National Programme has supported 700 centres of Nehru Yuvak Kendras financially in order to spread messages about Family Life Education, and responsible sexual behaviour among rural youth. Special workshops have been held in the North East region, which is especially vulnerable to drug abuse, to integrate the component of HIV/AIDS in education programmes. A number of multimedia workshops and cultural programmes using folk art forms such as puppet shows, magic shows, music and local dance forms are used to disseminate information on HIV/AIDS in the rural areas through the out-reach activities of these youth clubs.

Print Media

The IEC division of NACO has prepared several packages of materials aimed at various population groups, to be used by the out-reach workers, health workers and peer educators working in government as well as non-government organisations.

TARGETED INTERVENTIONS

Certain categories of people, who are at a higher risk of acquiring and transmitting HIV infection, also described as

"Core transmitters" assume importance in prioritising cost effective interventions to prevent HIV infection. The basic purpose of the Targeted Intervention programme is to reduce the rate of transmission among the most vulnerable and marginalised populations. One of the ways of controlling the disease from further spread is to carry out direct intervention programmes among these groups through multi-pronged strategies, beginning from behaviour change communications, counselling, providing health care support, treatment for STDs and creating an enabling environment that will facilitate behaviour change. Targeted intervention is, therefore, one of the most important components of the NACP-II.

It envisages a comprehensive and integrated approach to marginalised and vulnerable populations such as sex workers, intravenous drug users, men having sex with men, truckers, migrant labour and street children. Since majority of these groups are marginalised both, socially and economically, it is not possible to access them through conventional Government services. NGOs, Community based Organisations and other appropriate agencies are able to reach out to these populations more effectively. These groups need information and services in a focused and non-judgmental manner. It is, therefore, important to develop a pear-based approach, which enables and sustains behaviour change. These interventions must be supported by an environment that is conducive to empowering them for behaviour change. The Targeted Intervention approach, as defined by NACO, incorporates all the above components to provide comprehensive interventions in the marginalised groups to reduce the rate of transmission of the STDs and HIV infections. In order to plan for implementation of this programme NACO evolved the following strategy.

i) Decentralisation of implementation to the State AIDS Control Society.

ii) Transparent and streamlined procedures for selection of NGOs.

iii) Capacity building of SACS and NGOs for implementation and monitoring of TI Projects.

Implementation

The State AIDS Control Societies are fully empowered to provide funding support to the NGOs for initiating Targeted Interventions. Every State AIDS Control Society has appointed an NGO Advisor, who is a professional in the field of social work, to manage and guide the Targeted Intervention Programme. Detailed guidelines have been formulated by NACO for the short-listing of local NGOs and for their training and orientation in Targeted Interventions.

NACO had conducted two rounds of intensive training programmes for the officers of the State AIDS Control Societies to empower them in supporting the programme on Targeted Interventions effectively. The five-day training programmes were held in Delhi and were attended by these officers, including the Project Director and NGO Advisor from the State AIDS Control Society.

A training module was developed in collaboration with UNAIDS and distributed to all the States for conducting training programmes for NGOs. In order to ensure cost effective and comprehensive Targeted Interventions, NACO has formulated a costing pattern for each of the Targeted Interventions in the identified marginalised group. This costing pattern was developed after participatory discussions with agencies who have implemented Targeted Interventions successfully in the country. This costing pattern provides a guiding framework to the states in sanctioning projects. The Targeted interventions are being monitored and evaluated regularly to ensure that the maximum impact is created at the grass root level. Almost 554 TI projects have been undertaken by the State AIDS Control Societies through NGOs in different locations in the country.

CSW Interventions	132
Truckers Interventions	127
Migrant workers Interventions	185
IDU Interventions	35
Street Children Interventions	28
MSM Interventions	17
Prison inmates Interventions	30

More than 50 per cent of the total TI Projects are in the high prevalent states like Andhra Pradesh, Maharashtra, Tamil Nadu, Karnataka, Manipur and Nagaland.

Control of Sexually Transmitted Disease (STD)

There is enough evidence to suggest that STDs, particularly those characterised by genital ulcers, increase the chance of HIV infection. This highlights the need for concomitant control of STDs as a programme strategy. The STD control component of the National AIDS Control Programme has two major objectives:

i) Reduce STD cases and there by control HIV transmission by minimising the risk factor and;
ii) Prevent the short term as well as long term morbidity and mortality due to STD.

The five regional STD Reference Laboratories have been upgraded to provide necessary training for doctors and laboratory technicians on STD diagnosis and management. During the year, 5 regional level training programmes were conducted for the Microbiologists and separately for the technicians on the diagnosis of STDs. STD clinics functioning in districts medical colleges have been strengthened and doctors trained on the Syndromic management of STDs. It has been observed that a large number of female patients of STD attend the gynaecology clinics for treatment.

A comprehensive training programme conducted for the gynaecologists on a regional basis at Safdarjung Hospital. New Delhi and other hospitals in the country were oriented to treat the STDs and reproductive tract infections (RTIs) within their settings rather than referring to STD clinics. Drugs for the treatment for the STDs/RTIs are being provided by the State AIDS Control, societies to all the STD clinics as well as the Gynaecology clinics.

In order to ensure complete and correct treatment, uniform guidelines and flowcharts have been distributed to all medical practitioners both in government hospitals and in private practice, thus minimising the chances of increasing drug resistance. However, there is a need to improve the quality of services in the STD clinics to attract more patients, particularly those seeking treatment through unqualified practitioners.

Condom Promotion

For the effective control of STDs and HIV/AIDS, the condom programme of NACO is an important strategy to combat the epidemic. The objectives of the condom programme is to ensure easy access to god quality, affordable and acceptable condoms to promote safe sexual encounters. Emphasis on this activity by NACO has led to:

i) Improved quality Control of Condoms
ii) Introduction of social marketing of Condoms
iii) Involvement of NGOs in the programme

The common approach for condom promotion include:

i) *Free supply distribution:* The Department of Family Welfare is promoting distribution of condoms under this scheme through the network of health infrastructure and functionaries working in hospitals/clinics/PHCs/CHCs/

SCs. There is also involvement of personnel of non-health departments like Anganwadi workers, school teachers etc.

ii) *Social marketing:* The department of Family Welfare has identified private marketing companies for the promotion of condoms under this scheme. The government provides condoms at highly subsidised price to the marketing companies and they in turn, distribute it to the States/ UTs through their marketing network. The retail outlet is the last outlet and the customer procures the product from the retail outlet. NACO has also introduced social marketing and 3.30 million pieces of Delux Nirodh were earmarked for the programme during the year 2000-2001. NGOs are being encouraged to undertake social marketing of condoms besides free distribution.

iii) *Commercial distribution:* Commercial condoms are predominantly sold through chemist outlets and departmental stores. The condoms produced at the manufacturing points are sent to state level distributors who distribute them to the districts and town stockists. They, in turn, send them to retail outlets.

Table 1
Distribution of condoms

Year	*Free distribution (in millions)*	*Social marketing (in millions)*
1995-96	891.22	162.92
1996-97	685.85	263.25
1997-98	741.70	324.42
1998-99	660.76	348.74
1999-2000	674.36	348.74
2000-2001	627.42	465.43

Source: Deptt. of family welfare, Govt. of India

Family Health Awareness Campaign

The importance of Reproductive Tract infections (RTI) including sexually transmitted diseases (STD) has increased with the introduction of HIV/AIDS epidemic in the country. Early diagnosis and effective treatment of RTI/STD can significantly reduce transmission of HIV/AIDS. The Family Health Awareness Campaign is an effort to address the key issues related to reproductive health in the country, especially in rural and marginalised population. Four rounds of Family Health Awareness Campaigns have been conducted through out the country from 1999 to 2001. The last round of the Family Health Awareness Campaign was conducted during the period April to June, 2001. The period of the campaign was 15 days and was decided by the States as per their convenience. The objectives of the campaign were:

i) To raise the awareness levels regarding HIV/AIDS in rural and slum areas and other vulnerable groups of the population;

ii) To make people aware about the services available under the public sector for management of RTI/STD;

iii) To facilitate early detection and prompt treatment of RTI/STD cases by utilising the infrastructure available under primary health care system, including provision of drugs;

iv) To strengthen the capacity of medical and paramedical professionals working under health care system to respond to HIV/AIDS epidemic adequately. For the effective coordination and implementation of the campaign, Coordination Committees at State level under the Chairpersonship of Chief Secretary and District Coordination Committees under the Chairpersonship of District Magistrate were constituted. Comprehensive guidelines were given to the states and additional funds were provided for conduction of the campaign.

Prevention of Mother to Child transmission of HIV

The transmission efficiency of mother—to—child transmission of HIV infection ranges from 13-60 per cent. With increasing HIV infection among antenatal women in certain high prevalent states, paediatric AIDS is poised to become an important public health problem. The PACTG 076 trial offered Zidovindine (AZT) to HIV infected pregnant women between 14-34 weeks of gestation orally till delivery and intravenously during labour and also newborns for 6 weeks post-natally, reduced transmission of HIV-1 by 67 per cent. This led to the recommendation to use AZT in HIV infected women in the US as a public health policy. Report of about 50 per cent reduction in MTCT of HIV-1 from a collaborative study conducted in Thailand where AZT was administered after 36 weeks of gestation to the mother in the dosage of 300 mg twice a day and 300 mg every three hours during delivery increased the feasibility of extending this short course Thai regime in other developing countries including India.

A pilot study on Prevention of Mother to Child Transmission (MTCT) was initiated in 11 centres in India from January 2000. The enrolment of patients was initiated in March 2000.

1) Sir. J.J. Group of Hospitals , Mumbai
2) KEM Hospital, Mumbai
3) BYL Nair Hospital, Mumbai
4) General Hospital, Sanglli, Maharashtra
5) B.J. Medical Collage & Sasson Hospital, Pune
6) Government RSRM Hospital, Chennai
7) Kasturba Gandhi Hospital, Chennai
8) Institute of Obstetrics & Gynaecology, Egmore, Chennai
9) Osmania Medical Collage, Hyderabad, Andhra Pradesh
10) Banglore Medical Collage, Banglore, Karnataka
11) J.N. Medical Collage, Imphal, Manipur.

The objective was primarily to assess the feasibility of administration of AZT to prevent mother-to- child transmission of HIV-1 infection in pregnant mothers. All pregnant women attending the antenatal clinics in these institutions are offered a HIV group education-cum-counselling session supported by a video film session. At the end of the session, the participants are offered HIV test. Written informed consent is obtained from the women and blood sample for HIV test is collected. The post test counselling is offered on one-to-one basis. Women giving consent are enrolled in the study. All routine clinical and laboratory examination are conducted. Following exclusion criteria are used while screening these pregnant women;

i) Women attending hospital for the first time in labour
ii) Receipt of anti-retroviral therapy in last 2 months.
iii) Women attending clinic but planning delivery elsewhere.
iv) Women with major systemic disease or life threatening disorder.
v) Women severely anaemic (Hb< 8gm per cent)
vi) Women with severe mental abnormality.

After 12 weeks of gestation, the mothers are given Vitamin A 25000 IU weekly till delivery. From 36 weeks of gestation, AZT 300 mg orally twice a day is administered. During labour AZT 300 mg orally is given every 3 hours. However, no anti-retroviral drug is given to the infant. A PCR test is done at 48 hours and at 2 months of age for the determination of the HIV status of the infant. The option of breast feeding is left to the mother to decide after counselling on the risks and benefits of various option of infant feeding practices. This study has completed one year on 31st March 2001 and the results are being analysed for its operational feasibility, and efficacy, and also for various other related issues like acceptability of HIV testing, counselling and breast feeding etc. The achievements under the project till March 31, 2001 are as follows:

Total antenatal clinic attendees	1,52,376
No. of mothers counselled	1,20,363 (79 per cent)
No. of mothers accepted HIV test	92,838 (77.1 per cent)
No. of Mothers detected HIV positive	1704 (1.8 per cent)
No. of mothers delivered with AZT	640
per cent of babies PCR positive at 48 hours	49 (7.6 per cent)
per cent of babies PCR positive at 2 months	30 (9.7 per cent)

A feasibility study of single dose Nevirapine intervention is being planned by NACO in all the above 11 centres, which participated in conducting AZT feasibility study, and will be operational from 1st October 2001. A single dose of 200 mg of Nevirapine will be administered to the mother during the first stage of labour and single dose of 2 mg/kg body weight to the new born within 72 hrs. of birth in mothers who volunteer to enrol themselves in the study.

Limited studies have shown the potential benefit of post-exposure prophylaxis to health care workers following exposure to infection due to a needle-stick or sharp injury. Though the risk and acquiring HIV infection during occupational exposure is low (0.3 per cent), health care setting, improvement of hospital infection control practices and adoption of standard safety precautions can further reduce the risk. With the introduction of anti-retroviral drugs for post-exposure prophylaxis, the fear of occupational exposure among health care workers while managing HIV/AIDS patients is gradually diminishing and more and more doctors are motivated in treating these patients. NACO has made provisions for 2-3 anti-retroviral drugs to be made available to the staff in all medical institutions. Since these drugs have to be monitored for its toxicity and side effects, NACO insists on a registry to be maintained in all these hospitals for information on the number of occupational exposures and health workers sero-converting due to such an exposure. At present, only one nursing staff has been reported to have become HIV positive due to occupational exposure in India.

CARE FOR HIV/AIDS PATIENTS

Over the years, there has been a steady increase in the number of AIDS cases seeking treatment in various hospitals across the country. A cumulative total of 20,304 cases of AIDS had been reported to the National AIDS Control organisation (NACO) till 31st March 2001. With an estimated number of 3.86 million HIV infections in the country, the number of AIDS cases is likely to continue to increase in the coming years. Realising the enormity of the situation, NACO has accorded a high priority to provide optimal care and support to HIV infected persons. Various activities of NACO initiated in the second phase of the programme aim at providing quality clinical management of cases in hospitals besides providing psychosocial support to the individuals and their families. Some of the important activities are discussed below.

Training

Though training has been an ongoing activity of NACO, newer areas of management and hospital infection control measures including post-exposure prophylaxis necessitate the need for periodic training and orientation with updated information and guidelines. The programme training has been structured in different tiers, with comprehensive curriculum for different categories of the health functionaries. The objective is to involve all the medical, paramedical and field staff and attain complete coverage by March 2002. However, by the end of March 2001 the following coverage has been achieved :

Total Number of Doctors trained	24,153
Total number of Nurses trained	26,607
Total number of other paramedical workers	27,688

These figures include 1830 Core trainers in all the states/UTs. These core trainers, ten in each medical college and other tertiary hospital, are responsible for imparting training to the District level core trainers and also to their colleagues and other staff in their institutions. Most of the states have completed this training in the medical colleges. All the districts in the country have an identified district nodal officer. The training of these nodal officers have been covered in batches of 30 each and a multi-speciality District Training Team (DTT) has been identified and trained in most of the districts. However, the training of the paramedical staff and the staff in the Primary Health Centres (PHCs) need to be scaled up to meet the timeline of complete coverage by March 2002. The feedback from these training programmes have been encouraging. More number of doctors have started treating AIDS cases in their respective areas and the referral of cases to tertiary hospitals has been reduced considerably.

In order to sensitise the Deans and the Medical Superintendents of the medical colleges towards effective implementation of care and support and hospital infection control practices, three regional workshops were organised in Delhi on the 15th of February & 3rd of April 2001 and in Patna on the 23rd of May 2001. These programmes were well attended and the participants deliberated on various issues related to clinical management of AIDS cases in hospitals. Besides, the Medical Council of India agreed to include HIV/AIDS in the undergraduate and postgraduate courses. The salient recommendations from these workshops were :

i) Voluntary Counselling & Testing Centres (VCTC)
   a) VCTCs may be located near Out Patients Departments (OPDs) for better access
   b) Linkages may be developed between VCTC, STD clinics, medicine OPD, antenatal clinics and blood banks

ii) Each institution must have a Hospital Infection Control Committee and meetings should be conducted periodically. A quarterly report on needle stick exposures and Post Exposure Prophylaxis (PEP) may be sent to NACO/SACS.

iii) The Department of Microbiology may be considered as the nodal department for HIV/AIDS activities including reporting to NACO.

iv) A comprehensive training workshop on Hospital Infection Control may be taken up by States.

v) Some of the medical colleges may be identified as centres of excellence for hands-on training on HIV/AIDS case management.

vi) Data from sentinel surveillance should be disseminated to the individual medical institutions for their information.

vii) Introduction of HIV/AIDS in undergraduate and postgraduate curriculum may be implemented and all the medical colleges/universities may be intimated in this regard.

Overall, these training programmes have led to better management of AIDS cases in hospitals, improvement in hospital infection control practices and ownership of the programme at institutional level.

Voluntary Counselling and Testing

HIV voluntary counselling and testing (VCT) has been shown to play an important role in both HIV prevention and care as an entry point. It provides people with an opportunity to learn and accept their HIV serostatus in a confidential enabling environment. VCT has become an integral part of HIV prevention programmes in many countries, as it is a relatively cost-effective intervention in preventing HIV transmission. The potential benefits of VCT are:

i) Better ability to cope with HIV-related anxiety

ii) Motivation to initiate or maintain safer sexual practices

iii) Motivation to change drug related behaviour
iv) Prevention of HIV-related illnesses
v) Early access to care and support
vi) Improved Health status through good nutritional advice
vii) Emotional Support
viii) Awareness about safer options for reproduction and infant feeding
ix) Safer blood donation

Currently, there are 142 Voluntary Counselling and Testing Centres located in the microbiology departments. Majority of the VCTCs are established in medical colleges and tertiary care hospitals. The expansion of this programmatic component in the next couple of years will ensure establishment of one VCTC in each district hospital in the high HIV prevalence States. As an entry point to care and support services for HIV/AIDS, the VCTCs are well equipped with diagnostic facilities for HIV infection and provide counselling services through trained counsellors. The counsellors not only cater to patients who walk in but also to HIV/AIDS cases admitted in hospital and antenatal mothers. Besides ELISA facilities, rapid HIV diagnostic test kits are also provided to obtain test results in emergency and when the turnout of person requiring HIV tests is low in a VCTC.

An External Quality Assessment Scheme (EQAS) is also being introduced to ensure quality control in HIV testing laboratories.

Clinical Management of HIV/AIDS

Though there is gross under-reporting of full-blown AIDS cases, a total of 20,304 cases with various opportunistic infections have been reported to NACO till < 31st March 2001. The details of the AIDS cases are as follows:

Table 2

National AIDS control programme AIDS cases in India (As on 31st March, 2001)

S. No	*State / UT*	*AIDS Cases*
1.	Andhra Pradesh	612
2.	Assam	110
3.	Arunachal Pradesh	0
4.	A & N Islands	13
5.	Bihar	44
6.	Chandigarh (UT)	292
7.	Delhi	500
8.	Daman & Diu	1
9.	Dadra & Nagar Haveli	0
10.	Goa	29
11.	Gujarat	689
12.	Haryana	48
13.	Himachal Pradesh	85
14.	Jammu & Kashmir	2
15.	Karnataka	918
16.	Kerala	267
17.	Lakshadweep	0
18.	Madhya Pradesh	664
19.	Maharashtra	4459
20.	Orissa	55
21.	Nagaland	103
22.	Manipur	790
23.	Mizoram	16
24.	Meghalaya	8
25.	Pondicherry	141
26.	Punjab	131
27.	Rajasthan	272
28.	Sikkim	2
29.	Tamilnadu	9714
30.	Tripura	0
31.	Uttar Pradesh	282
32.	West Bengal	57
	Total:	**20304**

People living with HIV/AIDS experience a variety of health and social support needs as their illness progresses and opportunistic infections occurs. For the clinical management of these cases certain policies and guidelines have been developed. They are as follows:

i) All the Government hospitals have been instructed to admit HIV/AIDS cases without any discrimination. They have to be managed in the general wards of the hospitals along with other patients except cases having sputum positive (open) pulmonary tuberculosis and when the patient's immunity is completely diminished. This is required to protect him from other infections and thus he needs to be managed in a separate room. Any special marking or board near the beds for HIV positive patients is discouraged.

ii) The discharge certificate will only refer to their opportunistic infection from which they suffer. Mention about their HIV status on their discharge certificate is discouraged. Only the case sheet should contain the diagnosis of HIV/AIDS. Similarly in death certificates, only the immediate cause of death that is the primary cause or opportunistic infection will be mentioned.

iii) It has been emphasised to all Project Directors of State AIDS Control Societies to ensure that patients of HIV/AIDS admitted in general hospital should get drugs for opportunistic infection free of cost. All the Project Directors of State/UT AIDS Control Societies should provide funds for treatment of opportunistic infections to the Superintendents of Government hospitals upto the district levels depending upon the number of AIDS cases treated by then during the previous years. It should be ensured that all opportunistic infections are treated properly. HIV-infected tuberculosis patients should be treated according to the RNTCP guidelines by the local tuberculosis officer.

iv) Infection Control guidelines in the government hospitals should be followed strictly. All tertiary care and district hospitals should establish local infection control committee, which meets once a month. State AIDS Control Societies should motivate the state governments to ensure supply of equipment requitred in undertaking appropriate infection control measures in hospitals like incinerators, autoclaves etc. There should be no complacency over infection control measures. The State government should also ensure regular and adequate supplies of gloves, masks and other consumable items in hospitals for the protection of the health care workers for nosocomial infections.

v) Post exposure prophylaxis should be strictly monitored and two doses of PEP drugs are kept with the emergency medical officer to make them available whenever the need arises.

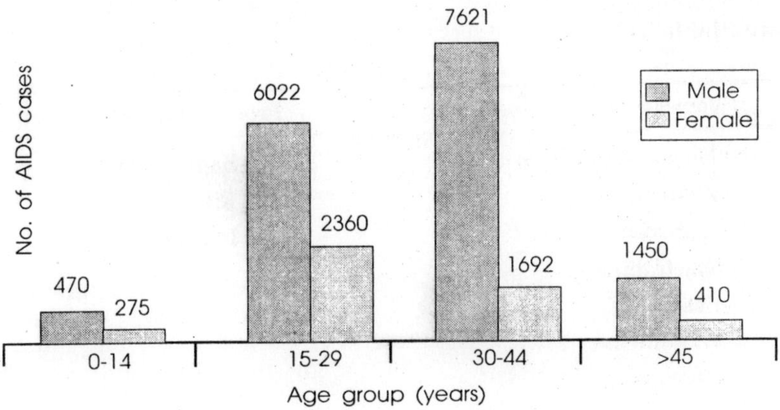

Figure 2: Age and sex distribution of reported AIDS Case in India (n = 20304) May 1986-March 2001)

As HIV/AIDS is a disease with long incubation period, there should be proper home care facilities. The home care should be delivered by NGOs/CBOs by establishing linkages with the

Community Health Care Projects and Health Centres. Family members should be taught to treat minor symptoms like cough, diarrhoea, fever and proper nursing care etc.

Anti-retroviral Therapy

Anti-retroviral drugs are agents that inhibit the replication of HIV in an infected person. These act on the various stages of life cycle of the virus. At present, there are 8 such anti-retroviral which are available in the country. These anti-retrovirals drugs remain to be out of reach of many due to high costs. However, there has been a dramatic reduction in prices of these drugs recently. Monitoring the patients on anti-retroviral drugs is an important aspect of anti-retroviral therapy which adds to the cost of total treatment. There are two groups of anti-retroviral drugs—Reverse Transcriptase Inhibitors which has two subgroups—Nucleoside Analogue and Non-nucleoside Analogue; and Protease Inhibitors. The drugs which are available in India are:

Reverse transcriptase inhibitors	*Protease inhibitors*
Nucleoside Analogue	Saquinavir
Zidovudine	Ritonavir.
Lamivudine	Indinavir.
Zalcitabine.	
Stavudine.	
Didanosine.	
Abacavir	
NonnucleosideAnalogue:	
Nevirapine	
Efavirenz	

Policy on Anti-retroviral therapy

NACO is making all efforts to exempt customs and excise duty on all Anti-retroviral drugs available in India in order to reduce their prices. The Anti-retroviral therapy for treatment of AIDS patients is not provided under the National Programme. However, in the training programmes for doctors the rationale use of Anti-retroviral therapy is emphasised. Anti-retroviral drugs are provided under the programme in cases of post-exposure prophylaxis to health care providers and the feasibility study project on prevention of mother to child transmission.

HUMAN RIGHTS, GENDER AND DISCRIMINATION

The HIV/AIDS epidemic is not merely a health issue but a development challenge that impacts the social, economic, cultural, political and legal parameters of society. The epidemic further aggravates the socioeconomic vulnerabilities of the weakest in society including women and children and marginalised groups which have little or no access to basic human rights such as food, medical services and information. Since many of these groups are ostracised by society and thus affecting their lifestyles adversely, it is difficult for them to participate in mainstream processes whereby they can demand their rights.

Global experience has demonstrated that the spread of HIV/AIDS is facilitated by human rights violations. These include gender disparities, absence of choices, lack of access to economic resources leading to migration or trafficking, denial of treatment and discrimination in health care and / or in the work place. These human rights violations often lead to the infection going underground and spreading even faster. In order to be effective, HIV/AIDS prevention and control strategies, specially in developing countries, need to address the issue of human rights violations and create an enabling environment that increases knowledge and encourages behaviour change. Access to voluntary counselling and testing needs to be promoted along with affordable care and support. In particular, the vulnerabilities of women and children due to social, cultural norms and diminishing opportunities to generate income from agriculture need to be addressed in a focused and sustainable manner.

NACO has adopted multipronged strategies to address the socioeconomic dimensions of the epidemic. The most important strategy among priority groups such as sex workers, truckers, men having sex with men, injecting drug users and migrants is targeted interventions. These interventions embody a comprehensive approach that combines behaviour change communication, provision of STD treatment and condoms along with the creation of enabling environment. The component of enabling environment is essential and critical to the success of Targeted Interventions. The activities undertaken under this component seek to identify and address the socioeconomic, cultural and legal barriers that prevent communities from adopting a safer lifestyle to protect themselves from HIV/AIDS. In many cases these activities go beyond the health sector and range from political advocacy, provision of basic civic amenities & care to protection for children. NGOs are involved in implementing the Targeted Intervention programmes since they have the necessary connectivity with the community and are able to establish appropriate channels of communication and mechanisms for community participation in the delivery of services. The Targeted Intervention approach, therefore, seeks to empower communities not only in the context of HIV/AIDS prevention, but in the wider definition of socioeconomic development and fulfillment of the basic human rights.

The right to information, which is also a basic human right is at the core of HIV/AIDS prevention and control. The National AIDS Control Organisation has developed partnerships with both-Government and Non Governmental Organisations and agencies, which have a credible presence in the social sector to disseminate preventive messages about HIV/AIDS and increase knowledge among vulnerable population groups in particular. The School Education Programme is an important strategy in reaching young people for life skills education and developing skills that help them resist peer pressure and imbibe a supportive attitude towards those already infected. This programme has been developed on the basis of a successful experiment undertaken in Maharashtra with an NGO-Sevadham Trust and UNICEF. A manual entitled "Learning for Life" has been developed in consultation with NCERT and UNESCO. The programme envisages training of teachers and students. It adopts an extracurricular approach to AIDS awareness. It is proposed that this programme shall be extended to cover 20 per cent of schools in the country during the current year (2001-2002) in low prevalence States while 100 per cent coverage in six high prevalence States in India..

With reference to women and children, NACO has undertaken a collaborative programme with the Department of Women and Children, Ministry of Human Resource Development to train Anganwadi Workers, the grass root functionary of the Integrated Child Development Scheme (ICDS). The ICDS workers are being trained and sensitised on the issue of HIV/AIDS and STDs through their ongoing training programmes. Special IEC material has also been developed for Anganwadi Workers.

Reduction of stigma and discrimination alongwith protection of human rights at workplace is priority area for the National AIDS Control Programme. Political advocacy at the level of Prime Minister has been initiated to develop partnerships with the business sector and the civil society to ensure a policy of non-discrimination in recruitment and during employment. NACO is also working closely with the International Labour Organisation (ILO) and the Ministry of Labour for a Code of Conduct at workplace. Special strategies for the unorganised labour, who do not have access to the social safety nets, are also being implemented. NACO is supporting the Department of Youth Affairs, Ministry of Human Resource Development to strengthen and expand the programme of empowering rural youth through the Nehru Yuvak Kendras and college youth through "University Talks AIDS Programme" in collaboration with National Service Scheme (NSS). The strategy integrates the issue of HIV/AIDS prevention approaches with the ongoing programmes and activities of the Nehru Yuvak Kendras and the NSS.

Care and support of those already infected and their families is an important part of the National AIDS Control Programme. Drugs required in management of opportunistic infections are provided free of cost in the public hospitals. Community Care Centres are being established through NGOs to provide low-cost care and psychosocial support to those who are infected by HIV and their families. Voluntary counselling and testing centres are being established in every district hospital to provide pre and post-test counselling and testing facilities in a confidential environment. Networks and self-help groups of people living with HIV/AIDS are being encouraged to take up the advocacy and counselling activities. It is envisaged that these strategies would help to create an environment with less stigma and discrimination and help to mainstream issue of HIV/AIDS with the other social issues.

In November 2000, NACO co-sponsored a National Conference on Human Rights and HIV/AIDS in partnership with the National Human Rights Commission, Lawyers Collective, United Nations Children Funds and the United Nations Joint Programme on HIV/AIDS. The two days conference brought together officers of the State Human Rights Commissions, activists, NGOs and health officials to deliberate upon the issue of protection of human rights in the context of HIV/AIDS. The national consultation has given detailed recommendations on the subject which are under consideration of the Government.

QUALITY ASSESSMENT SCHEME FOR HIV TESTING

HIV infection can be diagnosed by the demonstration of specific antibodies and / or detection of viral antigens or RNA. However, ELISA or Rapid tests for detecting the antibodies against HIV are used predominantly. NACO has undertaken a massive expansion of the testing facilities upto the district level with the launching of VCTCs in all the districts in a phased manner. A high degree of concordance in test results between the HIV testing laboratories is one of the essential requirements for quality assurance of HIV testing.

Quality control is the sum of all activities and procedures undertaken by medical laboratories to improve the quality and clinical usefulness of laboratory test results. It has two components, external and internal. Internal quality control is the set of procedures employed by laboratory staff for continuous monitoring at the time of testing. This is inbuilt into the testing procedure.

External Quality assessment is undertaken to standardise the performance of laboratories with respect to each other. It is complimentary to internal quality control. The National AIDS Control Organisation has initiated the External Quality Assessment Scheme (EQAS) for all its HIV testing laboratories in a phased manner. The laboratories have been classified into different tiers which is as follows:

Phase I: In the first phase of the scheme the 12 National Reference laboratories participated in the programme in December 2000-January 2001. In this process a network was developed between the 12 laboratories. The sera panels for proficiency testing was developed by NIB and distributed to all the 12 laboratories. The results of the programme showed 100 per cent concordance.

Phase II: Of the scheme will involve the state reference laboratories (VCTCs located in the medical colleges and other tertiary hospitals) and the national reference laboratories. Each National Reference Laboratories was assigned some state VCTCs for quality control. As a first step, the microbiologists and the technicians involved in HIV testing were imparted training on EQAS. This programme is scheduled to be conducted during the months of September-October 2001, during the ongoing sentinel surveillance.

Phase III: This phase will involve the quality assurance of district VCTCs and the blood banks and is slated to be conducted in August –September, 2002.

It is envisaged that the EQAS will be conducted twice a year and as the programme continues, the laboratories will improve and the degree of variability will diminish. It would also be useful to pick out weak performers and help them achieve a standard bench mark.

PROGRAMME FINANCING

The IX Five Year Plan allocated an amount of Rs.760 crores for Prevention and Control of AIDS in India against the total cost of Rs.1155 crores. The balance amount will spill over to the first two years of the X Five Year Plan period. The allocation of funds for various components of the World Bank assisted NACP-II of Rs.1155 crore (World Bank and Govt. of India) is as follows:

Table 3

S.No	*Components*	*Outlay (Rupees in Crores)*
1	Prevention among High Risk Groups	265.60
2	Prevention among low risk groups	389.10
3	Care HIV/AIDS	163.30
4	Institutional Strengthening	286.50
5	Intrsectoral Collaboration	50.60

The amounts projected in the EFC Memorandum, budget estimates and its utilisation for National AIDS Control Programme—Phase II from 1999-2000 onwards are indicated below:

Table 4

(Rupees in crores)

Year	*Budget Estimate*	*Revised Estimate*	*Expenditure incurred*	*Percent utilisation*
1999-2000	140.00	140.00	135.25	96.60
2000-2001	145.00	180.00	179.00	123.45
2001-2002	210.00			

The implementation of the National AIDS Control Programme in India has been facilitated by the World Bank by providing a Credit of US$ 191 million. The Scheme though approved in September 1999 could be effectively implemented only from November 1999 onwards. The Agreement with the World Bank stipulated that Government of India would advance funds for the implementation of the Scheme to the States/Union Territories AIDS Control Societies as well as other implementing agencies and claim reimbursement from the World Bank by filing reimbursement claims on the basis of actual expenditure. Withdrawal of funds from the World Bank (IDA) Credit account has to be on the basis of actual expenditure incurred by NACO as well as each AIDS Control Society implementing this project.

The AIDS –II Project has been made effective from 9th November 1999 and a Special Account amounting to US $ 10.00 million has been maintained in the Reserve Bank of India. The Department of Economic Affairs of Govt. of India on the basis of Reimbursement claims filed under the project would operate this account. As on 31st March 2001 claims for Rs.141.57 crores have been sent to World Bank through Ministry of Finance, Department of Economic Affairs against which reimbursement of Rs.127.81 crores (US $ 41.364 Million) has been received.

AIDS Prevention and Control (APAC) Project in Tamil Nadu aims at tackling HIV transmission in State of Tamil Nadu by reinforcing HIV prevention behaviour among population at risk to the infection notably commercial sex workers and their clients and STD patients. The total commitment for this project is US $ 10 million or say Rs.30 crores in terms of Indian Rupees. By the end of 31st March 2001. Rupees 21.48 crores has been utilised under the Project. The USAID funded AVERT Project seeks to increase the use of effective and sustainable responses to reduce transmission of and mitigate STD/HIV/AIDS and related infectious diseases in the State of Maharashtra. A nodal agency to implement the Project has been established and a provision of Rs.7 crores has been kept for the current financial year.

Department for International Development (DFID) of UK is supporting a project for prevention and control of HIV/AIDS and other Sexually Transmitted Diseases in the State of Andhra Pradesh, Gujarat, Kerala and Orissa. The Project is adopting the same targeted Intervention approach in dealing with the vulnerable communities such as sex workers, intravenous drug users, prison inmates, street children and migrant workers as in the World Bank assisted National AIDS Control Project – Phase II. During 2000-2001 funds to the extent of Rs.8.00 crores have already been released. During the current financial year a provision of Rs.25 crores has been kept.

TECHNICAL RESOURCE GROUPS

Prevention and control of HIV/AIDS requires a multi-sectoral approach addressing various issues such as blood safety, prevention and control of sexually transmitted diseases, condom promotion, clinical management, protecting the rights of the HIV infected persons, etc. One of the important features of the present programme over that in Phase I is to obtain technical inputs from centres of excellence in various fields connected with prevention and control of AIDS and integrate them into the programme. It was thought that instead of providing a number of technical experts at the head quarter of NACO, it would be more cost-effective if the expertise available in various institutions in the country is utilised for obtaining necessary technical inputs for the programme. Constitution of Technical Resource Groups (TRGs) is a critical component of the IInd phase of the programme. Certain thematic areas have been identified to constitute Technical Resource Groups (TRGs) in various institutes of excellence in the country. In view of the experience gained in last 2 years on the functioning of TRGs, it was felt necessary to examine the gaps in the present activities of the TRGs and identify necessary steps to be taken for effective functioning of TRGs. Following a series of meetings with TRG Chairs, Coordinators, TRG members and members of

SACS; certain guidelines were provided to TRGs in order to ensure clarity in terms of institutional arrangement, terms of reference, composition of TRG, and support mechanism etc. Based on these recommendations, following guidelines are issued for streamlining of TRG process under the National AIDS Control Programme:

— Institutional arrangement
— Criteria for the institution that hosts the TRG will be as follows:
— The theme of the institute should be directly related to the functioning of the TRG
— The institute should be willing to provide an expert faculty from within who shall spend a significant amount of time with the TRG work.
— The institution should be willing to abide by the norms spelt out by NACO from time to time.
— The institution should have a thematic mandate for HIV
— The institution should have a long term programmatic perspective
— Space, personnel and functional autonomy to be provided by the institute.

To assist the National AIDS Control Organisation in implementing the Phase II of the National AIDS Control Programme by providing appropriate technical assistance as and when required. The identify the best practices nationally through systematic evaluation of the National AIDS Control Programme and globally through literature review. Identify the past successes and articulate the element and context of the success in the 'best practices document'. To devise appropriate TRG programme strategies in consonance with the three stages of the HIV epidemic and clearly develop a plan to offer complementary products and technical assistance to ensure effective delivery of National AIDS Control Programme in the States/UTs. To determine realistic goals and achievable programme goals in each programme component falling under the TRG over the next five years on a short-and-long-term basis. Identify the outcomes and end points for each goal along with the technical and human resources required to achieve them. To provide appropriate technical assistance to all the State AIDS Control Societies in India on both, "on demand" and 'proactive basis'. To devise strategies to facilitate interaction between the State AIDS Control Societies and UTs and the TRG on a regular basis. To develop appropriate quality guidelines, technical assistance products and training programmes using national, regional and global expertise through meetings including virtual meetings and the process of peer review.

INTERNATIONAL AND BILATERAL COOPERATION

A number of multilateral and bilateral development agencies are extending technical and financial support for implementation of projects for the prevention and control of HIV/AIDS in India. Working together with National AIDS programme, the Joint United Nations Programme on HIV/AIDS (UNAIDS) and its seven UN co-sponsor agencies UNICEF, UNDP, UNFPA, UNESCO, WHO, UNDCP and World Bank; are striving to combat the AIDS epidemic through concerted efforts.

World Health Organisation

WHO's major contribution has been in programme management, surveillance, STD control, blood safety and clinical management. United Nations Educational, Scientific and Cultural Organisation (UNESCO/ United Nations Population Fund (UNFPA) These agencies are assisting in school based AIDS education and non-student youth programmes. The UNFPA has been involved in integration of the HIV/AIDS programme with that of the Reproductive and Child Health (RCH) programme.

The International Labour Organisation has initiated a project for interventions in work place in collaboration with the Ministry of Labour and the National AIDS Control Organisation. The project envisages interventions both at the workplace and in communities of unorganised labour to create awareness, bring about behaviour change and encourage health-seeking behaviour through promotion of condoms and STD treatment. Other partners in the project are trade unions and employer associations. The World Bank is supporting the implementation of the programme since 1992.

United Nations International Children's Fund (UNICEF) Besides assisting in school based AIDS education programme, UNICEF is also supporting feasibility study on Prevention of Mother to Child Transmission (PMTCT) of HIV infection in 11 centres in India.

United Nations AIDS (UNAIDS): The goal of the integrated UN Work plan is to support a multisectoral response to HIV/AIDS epidemic, as per the overall objectives of the Government of India. UNAIDS provides the coordinating, facilitating and monitoring inputs for all the UN agencies activities. It supports the Technical Resource Groups (TRGs). Additionally, it is involved in disseminating best practices and establishing an information system linking the country within and also to global efforts trends of HIV/AIDS. Specific areas for strengthening and objectives of UN Integrated Work plan during the second phase of the project are listed below:

World advocacy: Promote and maintain HIV/AIDS related issues as a priority at the national and state levels. Sensitise decision-makers, programme planers and implementers on the issues related to the four cross-cutting themes and generate commitment that these will be incorporated in all areas of programming.

Surveillance: Strengthening national and state level capacity in surveillance and monitoring of the epidemic. Promote data collection on the factors related to risk vulnerability to the epidemic and the data's application for policy development, programming and evaluation for an expanded response to the epidemic.

Decentralisation: Strengthening the state level capacity in programming and management of HIV/AIDS prevention and care, particularly, difficult-to-reach and vulnerable populations. Reduce the vulnerability of marginalised population and to alleviate the impact of HIV/AIDS on them. HIV/AIDS prevention for young people in particular for youth from low socioeconomic strata, slums and rural areas. To reduce the vulnerability of youth to HIV/AIDS.

Impact reduction: Provide care, support and protection of human rights of people living with HIV/AIDS. Mitigate the adverse health and socioeconomic impact of HIV/AIDS epidemic.

Information exchange support: Improve access to and more effective use of information available on HIV/AIDS nationally and globally.

Technical resource groups: Facilitate the accessibility to technical resources to the State AIDS Control Societies. For this purpose 11 technical resource groups have been constituted by NACO in major thematic areas. They are:

i) Blood Safety
ii) Clinical management,
iii) TB and Hospital Infection Control
iv) Counselling
v) Epidemiology
vi) Injecting Drug users
vii) Prevention at Workplace
viii) Research & Development
ix) STD & Condom Programme
x) Target Interventions
xi) Women and Children.

In the past years several Bilateral Agencies have shown their interest and have come up with encouraging support to the national effort for prevention and control of HIV/AIDS in India. Following are some of the major contributions made by such agencies.

The USAID funded $ 10 million AIDS Prevention And Control Project (APAC), currently operational in Tamil Nadu is being implemented through a Tripartite Agreement between the Government of India represented by NACO, United States Agency for International (USAID), and Voluntary Health Services (VHS), Chennai. APAC Project, because of its excellence through technical expertise, has become a model for the ongoing as well as upcoming projects in the country, in the arena of creating awareness about HIV/AIDS, and, taking preventive control measures on the spread of HIV infection. This success has been achieved through concerted efforts from a number of associated NGOs actively involved in the process. The AVERT project in Maharashtra is being implemented with an objective to increase the use of effective and sustainable response to reduce transmission of STD/HIV/AIDS and related infectious diseases. An amount of US $ 41.5 million is earmarked for this project. The components are as follows:

i) Intervention in sex industry;

ii) Improving Comprehensive health services;

iii) Reduce High Risk Behaviour in Priority Population

iv) Developing capacity of CBO/NGOs to respond effectively to STD/HIV/AIDS;

v) To develop Communications support Programmes;

vi) Improve Access, Availability and Use of Condoms in the Sex industry;

vii) Establish Pilot/Demonstration Programmes for Out-of-School Youth;

viii) To strengthen State and Municipal Capacity for Planning, Monitoring, and Evaluation of State and Municipal Programmes;

ix) To develop longer term HIV/AIDS Programme of Research and Surveillance in Maharashtra.

The Department for International Development, UK (DFID) is providing financial support of 1.5 million pound sterling for the "Sexual Health Project" in West Bengal, over a period of three years. The focus of activity of this project is to control programmes and develop IEC techniques. DFID is also supporting a national Healthy Highways Project with the truckers community.

The project is currently in the pilot phase and is proposed to be integrated into the NACP-II. In addition DFID has formulated "partnership for sexual health" project for the prevention and control of HIV/AIDS and other sexually transmitted infections in Andhra Pradesh, Gujarat, Kerala and Orissa for a five years at a total cost of Rs.154 crores of which Rs. 104.01 crores will be routed through GOI as local cost and Rs.50.29 crores as technical cost to be managed by DFID for this project: The objectives of the project are:

i) To ensure better sexual health for people vulnerable to sexually transmitted diseases (STDs) and HIV, especially the poor;
ii) Lowering incidence of sexually transmitted infections in the four states.

The components of the project are:

i) Surveillance;
ii) Condom programming by ensuring that quality condoms are made available and acceptable to those who are vulnerable to STD/HIV through effective social marketing;
iii) To strengthen service providers to respond to clients' needs through targeted interventions for vulnerable groups, such as sex workers and their clients, men having sex with men, migrant workers and prison inmates.

The European union is supporting an NGO—the Lawyers' Collective, for a project that aims at advocacy and law and to protect the human rights of those infected and/or affected by the AIDS epidemic.

The Government has approved the Canada-India Collaborative HIV/AIDS Project with a total budget of Rs.37.81 crores as part of the ongoing schemes of the NACP-II. The five-year project will provide specific support to the States of Karnataka and Rajasthan. The main components for Karnataka include capacity building of the Karnataka State AIDS Control Society and their implementing partners at the state level and implementation of a high quality demonstration project at the district level. In Rajasthan, the activities are capacity-building and implementation and rigorous evaluation of novel high quality demonstration projects in two communities i.e. rural migrant women and cast based sex workers.

HIV ESTIMATES FOR YEAR 2001

The annual round of HIV Sentinel survey was conducted in 320 sites in all the States and Union Territories during August-October 2001. The sites include 135 sites in STD clinics, 170 sites in Antenatal Clinics, 13 sites for IDUs and 2 sites for MSM. Based on the HIV prevalence rates in various risk groups, the number of HIV infections was estimated at the national level. In 1998, 1999 & 2000, while making the estimates, certain assumptions were taken into consideration.

These assumptions had evolved on the basis of consultation with a group of experts including eminent Epidemiologists and Bio-statisticians in the country as well as from WHO and UNAIDS. Based on these assumptions and consistent methodology, a similar worksheet was developed using 2001 HIV sentinel data. This worksheet was examined by a small working group of experts and subsequently discussed by the members of the 'Task force on surveillance' including international experts from WHO and UNAIDS. As per the recommendations of this expert group, updating was made in the assumptions for HIV estimates 2001.

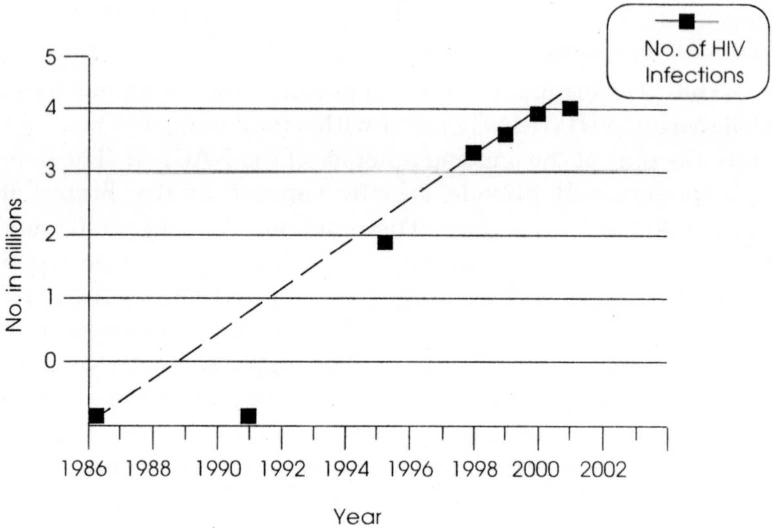

Figure 3: HIV estimates for year 2001

The point estimate for year 2001 comes to 3.31 million HIV infections in adult population (15-49 yrs. age group) in the country. With a 20 per cent variability to take care of unaccounted numbers of IDUs, MSM & other age groups, a working estimate of 3.97 million HIV infections was arrived at. The estimates for 1998,1999 and 2000 were 3.5 million infections, 3.7 million infections and 3.86 million infections respectively. The number of new infections can therefore be put at 0.11 million (3.97 - 3.86) in 2001 as compared to 0.16 million (3.86 – 3.7) in 2000. This shows that while the epidemic still spreading in the country, there is a gradual decrease in new infections.

Over a period of time, the new infections may reduce to a negligible number, which is an indicator of the plateauing of the epidemic. The existing indicators shows that such a phenomena may occur in next 3-4 year if a strong and effective programme is implemented in all the States/Union territories. This also indicates that in the north region of the country where the epidemic is still at low level, the focus should be to keep the epidemic at a low level.

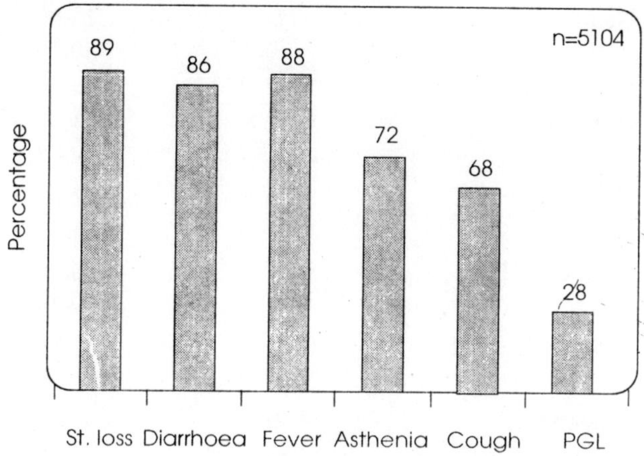

Figure 4: Epidemics level in India, 2001

States where the HIV prevalence in antenatal women is less than 1 per cent and HIV prevalence among STD and other high-risk group is less than 5 per cent.

Table 5

HIV Prevalence Levels State Wise : 2001

S.N.	*Name of State/UT*	*Number of Sites*	*HIV Prevalence 2001 (%)*
1.	Andhra Pd.	STD 4 ANC 9	26.60 1.50
2	Arunachal Pd.	STD 2 ANC 1	0.00 0.00
3	Assam	STD 2 ANC 3	1.49 0.00
4	Bihar	STD 5 ANC 7	1.20 0.13
5	Chattisgarh	STD 3 ANC 5	1.40 0.33

Contd...

6.	Delhi	STD 4	4.65
		ANC 4	0.13
		IDU 1	—
7	Goa	STD 2	15.00
		ANC 2	0.50
		CSW 1	50.79
8	Gujarat	STD 8	4.14
		ANC 7	0.50
9	Haryana	STD 4	1.08
		ANC 3	0.41
10	Himachal Pd.	STD 5	0.26
		ANC 7	0.13
11	Jammu & Kashmir	STD 2	0.80
		ANC 3	0.25
12	Jharkhand	STD 3	0.25
		ANC 6	0.08
13	Karnataka	STD 7	16.40
		ANC 10	1.13
		IDU 1	2.00
14	Kerala	STD 3	6.42
		ANC 3	0.08
15	Madhya Pd.	STD 6	2.69
		ANC 10	0.25
16	Maharashtra & Mumbai	STD 9	9.20
		ANC 14	1.75
		IDU 1	41.38
		MSM 1	23.60
		CSW 1	52.26
18	Manipur	IDU 3	56.26
		STD 2	1.75
		ANC2	10.50
19	Meghalaya	IDU 1	1.39
		STD 2	0.00
		ANC 2	0.00
20	Mizoram	IDU 1	2.00
		STD 2	2.20
		ANC 3	0.33

Contd...

21	Nagaland	IDU 2	5.50
		STD 1	7.40
		ANC 4	1.25
22	Orissa	STD 7	0.80
		ANC 4	0.25
23	Punjab	STD 3	1.61
		ANC 4	0.40
24	Rajasthan	STD 6	4.00
		ANC 6	0.00
25	Sikkim	STD 1	0.00
		ANC 2	0.00
26	Tamil Nadu	STD 5	12.60
		ANC 10	1.13
		IDU 1	24.56
		MSM 1	2.40
27	Tripura	STD 1	3.20
		ANC 1	0.25
		IDU 1	—
28	Uttar Pd.	STD 10	0.90
		ANC 11	0.00
29	Uttranchal	STD 4	0.40
		ANC 2	0.00
30	West Bengal	STD 6	0.60
		ANC 8	0.13
		IDU 1	—
31	A &N Islands	STD 1	1.20
		ANC 3	0.16
32	Chandigarh	STD 2	3.78
		ANC 1	0.00
33	D & N Haveli	ANC 1	0.25
34	Daman & Diu	ANC 2	0.25
35	L'dweep	STD 1	—
		ANC 2	—
36	Pondicherry	STD 3	2.00
		ANC 1	0.25

The justification for urban-rural and male-female gradient is as follows:

i) It is assumed that HIV spreads from urban to rural area and this differential is maintained even at very high level of HIV prevalence.

ii) It is assumed that higher percentage of males have risk behaviour as compared to females in India . In the beginning of the epidemic, males outnumber females and ratio gets closer to 1 with the progression of the epidemic in general population. In all the South-Asian countries, males outnumber females and in a high prevalence country like Thailand and Combodia, this ratio is between 1.6:2.

iii) It is also assumed that the infection shifts from high-risk population to general population over a period of time. Therefore, all the States go through a stage of low and then concentrated and finally generalised epidemic in the absence of effective interventions.

REFERENCES

NACO, HIV /AIDS India Scenario, 2001.

________________ , Combating HIV/AIDS in India, 2000-2001.

UNAIDS Report on the Global HIV/AIDS Epidemic, 2002.

WHO's Report on HIV/AIDS in Asia and the Pacific region, 2001.

4

AIDS in Pakistan: A Brief Sketch

According to estimates of UNAIDS, there are about 75,000 HIV infected people in Pakistan. Although the number of so far registered HIV infected people is 1549 out of which 202 were found with AIDS, yet there is a large number of people, who could not be registered or found due to social norms and stigma on AIDS as product of the sin. Whereas over three million deaths in the world occurred in the year 2000 due to AIDS alone, the tilt of vulnerability to the virus is towards Asia especially the Sub-continent. Over 5.7 million HIV victims have been reported in this part of the world.

Statistics show that adults are the most vulnerable to HIV and AIDS but unfortunately in our part of the world preventive measures are not proving as fruitful as in the west. In fact there is a need to reinterpret the concepts about AIDS, educate the people about the preventive measure, restore confidence and hope in HIV carriers and make society to stop hating them. It is not mere sexual contacts but a good many people have been affected with HIV through means other than sexual relations. If we look at the world AIDS scenario the ratio of people carrying AIDS virus through blood transfusion, HIV effected needle, syringe, razor, body piercing instruments, from mother to child etc.

In Pakistan the ratio of people with HIV through means other than sexual contacts is about 30 per cent which is even more alarming. AIDS is incurable but a little change in habits can serve as cure. In 1987 the National AIDS Programme was set up and 1994 branches of the National Aids Programme (NAP), were set in the four provincial capitals with more keeping in view the fast spread of HIV in Pakistan due to a large number of HIV carriers deported from the gulf states following AIDS screening tests in the Gulf States. According to a report recently published by the Federal Ministry of Health, the first officially recognised case of AIDS in Pakistan was that of an African sailor who was diagnosed in 1986 and died in 1987. The first case in Pakistani citizen, believed to have become infected with HIV while outside of Pakistan, was in 1987 in Lahore.

The majority of cases identified in these early years from the coastal city of Karachi and most of these cases were found were among non-Pakistanis. It was then commonly believed that AIDS was an infection of foreigners and that Pakistanis could not acquire it due to their strong traditions. This widespread public belief was denied, however, when in 1988 a Pakistani husband, wife and their child were all found to have become infected. During 1990 to 1995 Pakistanis living or travelling abroad became infected with HIV and then returned to Pakistan. In 1993, the first recognised transmission of HIV infection through breastfeeding in Pakistan.

In the mid to late 1990's cases of HIV and AIDS increasingly began to appear among such as sex workers, drug abusers and jail inmates. During this stage of Pakistan's epidemic it was recognised that transport workers and migrant labourers were beginning to spread the infection along the principal trade routes within the country. In addition, it is thought that inadequate sterilisation techniques and inappropriate use of medical equipment contributed to the broadening epidemic during this period. According to NAP hetro-sexual transmission currently accounts for the majority of HIV cases (37 per cent), 18 per cent infection is through contaminated blood or blood products and injecting drug use, four per cent homosexual, two bisexual and mother to child transmission is 1.3 per cent. The transmission modes of over 30 per cent cases is unknown.

Over 87 per cent of the reported HIV cases in Pakistan have been detected in men. Most of those infected fall within the age of 20-40 years, though just 16 per cent are in the forties. HIV cases have all the provinces and primarily from major urban areas within these provinces. If we consider in terms of gender women are the most vulnerable because of the disadvantages experienced by women. Female CSWs and female migrant workers are often exploited and abused, and have little recourse due to their low social status and limitations in legal protection. According to an information delivered by Dr Shafiq 12 surveillance centres for the HIV, Hepatitis C and drugs have been set to test and sort out preventive measures in keeping with the social norms.

It was also informed, recently the NAP established 46 HIV/AIDS surveillance centres in major cities of Pakistan. However most of the centres are not fully operational and many suffer shortages of diagnostic kits for HIV and other STIs. At the present time centres are largely functioning as screening centres for blood specimens referred to them and or not operating as effective surveillance and reporting centres. But what is more important is change in the behaviour of people towards AIDS victims.

A level of public awareness is necessary to facilitate the development of effective intervention programmes, fight stigma and discrimination, and ensure the delivery of high quality of care to those who are infected. There is need that electronic media comes forward and plays its part in focusing on awareness raising activities on groups at special risk or who are especially vulnerable, but the information needs of the general public must also be addressed.

During the recent years it has also been found that Tuberculosis (TB) is re-emerging as alarming threat. Drugs used for the cure of malady are not proving fruitful. It is guessed that TB may coincide with AIDS as there is no foolproof diagnosing system in Pakistan. There is need to address the problem with effective measures.

SOCIO-ECONOMIC BACKGROUND

Bestowed with abundant natural resources, a productive agriculture sector, a dynamic business community, and a strategic location for trade, Pakistan has achieved considerable growth since its independence in 1947.

However, the development indicators still remain poor. Only 40 per cent of the population is literate, compared to an average of 49 per cent in South Asia and 53 per cent in low-income countries worldwide. Gender disparities in education remain significant with about only around 62 per cent of Pakistan's girls enrolled in school compared to 80 per cent of its boys.

In the health sector, immunisation rates of most groups of children over the past decade have doubled and there is a dramatic increase in the knowledge of family planning. However, the improvement of other health indicators has been slow. One in every 38 women dies from pregnancy-related causes. Infant mortality remains high at about 90 per 1,000 live births, compared with an average of 75 per 1,000 in South Asian countries and 68 per 1,000 in low-income countries worldwide.

Poverty is still endemic and about two-fifths of the population does not have access to safe drinking water. More than half the population has no access to sanitation. Pakistan's population growth rate of 2.6 per cent is among the highest in the world.

On October 12, 1999, the then Nawaz Sharif government was deposed by a bloodless military coupled by General Pervez Musharraf. The military government set out on an ambitious reform agenda to bring Pakistan onto a new path of improved governance, growth, and poverty reduction. In particular, the reform programme focused on improvements in governance; fiscal reform; an enabling environment for private sector activity; devolution of power to lower levels of government; and bringing poverty reduction and the plight of marginalised people to the forefront of the development agenda.

Pakistan's long-standing economic and social challenges include a fragile macroeconomic situation; endemic governance problems; slow progress on poverty reduction since the early 1990s due to slackening economic growth, poor social indicators, particularly among women and in rural areas; severe gender disparities; and rapid urbanisation and associated environmental stresses.

Low levels of education and poor health are limiting Pakistan's productivity and adversely affecting medium-term growth and poverty reduction prospects. Despite some improvements over the past decade, Pakistan's social indicators, particularly for women, fall well short of other countries at a comparable stage of economic development.

The government launched the Social Action Programme (SAP) in 1992 to expand and improve the delivery of social services in elementary education, primary health, population welfare, and rural water supply and sanitation. The World Bank is leading a multidonor financial assistance programme to support SAP and in 1994, approved a $200 million credit for the Social Action Programme Project (SAPP), followed in March 1998 by the Second Social Action Programme Project (SAPPII), which was supported with a $250 million credit.

The measured impact of SAP includes higher school enrolment for girls, particularly in rural areas, significantly increased immunisation of children, and increased awareness of family planning. Under SAPP II, the government is building on this initial progress to raise enrolment and literacy rates further, to provide adequate basic health care for rural areas, to reduce infant mortality, and to increase access to safe water and sanitation.

In addition to the support through SAP, the World Bank assists Pakistan's health and education sectors through the Northern Health and Northern Education projects respectively. The health project aims to improve health conditions, particularly for women and children, and reduce unwanted pregnancies in Pakistan's Northern Areas and Azad

Jammu and Kashmir (AJK) provinces. The education project aims at improving both the quality of education and access, especially for girls. It is expected to benefit more than one million elementary school aged children living in the disadvantaged and remote mountainous regions of Pakistan. Most programmes are being delivered through a community-based approach. These initiatives are all significant but the government has a long way to go still to give basic education and health the central role they play in reducing poverty and promoting economic growth.

Weak urban management and a rapidly rising urban population severely strain the quality of life in Pakistan's cities and towns. The growth of urban population, at about four per cent annually, has raised serious development and management challenges. Efficiency of delivery systems and improvements in services need priority attention. The government's recently launched Integrated Rural and Urban Development Programme (IRUDP) aims to provide some relief in the short term. In addition, the Government is proposing major institutional and financial reforms through the Devolution Plan, which has the potential to bring about significant improvements in the functioning of local-level institutions and the provision of municipal services.

Agriculture remains the single most important sector in Pakistan, providing some 47 per cent of total employment, 60 per cent of export revenues and 90-95 per cent of food security needs. Nevertheless the sector has not made the contribution to poverty reduction that might be expected. Revitalising agriculture and realising its vast potential is one of the current Government's highest priorities.

Almost all-surface water is contaminated by pollution from domestic and industrial waste and agricultural runoff. Water and wind erosion, salinisation, water logging, and overgrasing have degraded about 42 per cent of the land in Pakistan's four provinces. Air pollution levels are rising and are already above World Health Organisation standards in Pakistan's two largest cities, Karachi and Lahore. The social costs of environmental degradation are likely to be enormous, having impacts on health and productivity as well as future livelihoods.

HIV SITUATION

The first case of AIDS in a Pakistani citizen was reported in 1987 in Lahore. During the late 1980s and 1990s, it became evident that an increasing number of Pakistanis, mostly men, were becoming infected with HIV while living or travelling abroad. Upon their return to Pakistan, some of these men subsequently infected their wives who, in some cases, passed along the infection to their children. During the 1990s, cases of HIV and AIDS began to appear among groups such as commercial sex workers (CSWs), drug abusers and jail inmates. The increased rates of infection among these groups are assumed to have facilitated, at least to some extent, a further dissemination of HIV into the general population.

Like in most of the region, the estimated HIV prevalence remains low at about 0.06 per cent of the population. Cases have been reported from all provinces, but they appear to have been confined mainly to people engaged in high-risk behaviour. Most of the infected persons belong to the 20 to 49 years age group. Until 1993, most infections were detected among foreigners and in Pakistani citizens returning from abroad. Though heterosexual route is the most common, infection through contaminated blood and blood products and through IDU is also prevalent.

Since the official recognition of the first case in 1987, the number of officially reported HIV infections and AIDS cases has grown to 1699 (as of September 2000). Heterosexual transmission accounts for the majority (37 per cent) of reported HIV cases, with the next most frequent mode of transmission (18 per cent) being related to infection through contaminated blood or blood products. The remainder of the reported HIV cases are linked with infection through injecting drug use (4 per cent), homosexual or bisexual sex (6 per cent), and mother to child transmission (1.3 per cent). Transmission modes for 35 per cent of the reported HIV cases are unknown. Unfortunately, most observers believe that the number of reported cases represents only the 'tip of the iceberg', and that the number of actual cases may be far greater than official reports suggest.

While HIV prevalence appears to be low in Pakistan at present, the presence of a number of vulnerabilities and risky behavioural patterns suggest the need for urgent, prioritised, and coordinated action to curtail the emergence of a widespread epidemic. Poverty, genders inequalities and low levels of education and literacy all contribute to HIV vulnerability in Pakistan. Other, related factors that can increase vulnerability at the individual level include unemployment, social exclusion or marginalisation, physical and/or mental abuse, and gender-based discrimination.

Reasons for Vulnerability

Poverty: Is a major development concern in Pakistan, and may be an important facilitating factor in the further spread of HIV infection in the country. While estimates vary, recent documentation suggests that poverty is undeniably on the rise in Pakistan, and that there are at least 36 million people (or 6 million households) that fall below the poverty line (Towards a National Poverty Strategy in Pakistan, Planning Commission, Government of Pakistan, 1999). It is important to note that the poor suffer not just limitations in income; they also lack basic facilities and amenities, which allow for a full and meaningful existence. For instance, limitations in access to health and education limit their ability to find work, which in turn limits their ability to make improvements in their lives. Importantly, such limitations also increase the likelihood that those who are most vulnerable are the least able to protect themselves from HIV infection, and, once infected, are the least able to gain access to the health and social support that they need.

Gender inequalities: May also play a facilitating role in the further spread of HIV/AIDS in Pakistan. Pakistani women in general have lower socioeconomic status, less mobility and less decision-making power than do men, all of which contributes to their HIV vulnerability. For example, because of gender disparities in educational enrolment, the female literacy rate in Pakistan is much lower than that of males (35 per cent for women as compared to 59 per cent for men according to the Government of Pakistan's Economic Survey 1999-2000). Thus, while illiteracy presents an obstacle for HIV/AIDS prevention efforts in general, it is much harder to reach women than men with information about how they can protect themselves from HIV infection. Women also are under-represented in the formal labour force, which, combined with their lower literacy rate and educational levels, reinforces their economic and social dependency on men. Additionally, restrictions on mobility often make it difficult for women to obtain access to health and social services, including access to basic reproductive health care. Finally, in situations where their decision-making power is restricted, it is unlikely that all women are equipped with the skills necessary to negotiate with their partners for safer sexual practices.

Blood transfusion: The collection and transfusion of blood and blood products, the use and re-use of unsterilised medical instruments (especially needles and syringes) and the generally low level of attention to standard infection control procedures are important potential avenues for the spread of HIV in Pakistan's general population. The indiscriminate use of blood transfusions and of needles in both the formal and informal health sectors is common. In addition, standard procedures for infection control in health care settings are often not strictly followed. A relatively high prevalence of both hepatitis B and C infection in the general population suggests that unsafe blood transfusion practices and poor infection control are likely to make a significant contribution to the further rapid spread of these infections and of HIV/AIDS among the general population.

Commercial sex workers: Some individuals and groups of people are especially vulnerable to HIV/AIDS due to their social status, particular behaviour patterns, or other special characteristics. For instance, the social and economic disadvantages experienced by women in Pakistan sometimes results in their involvement in livelihood strategies, which enhance their vulnerability to HIV and other STIs. Female commercial sex workers (CSWs) and female migrant workers are often exploited and abused, and have little recourse due to their low social status and limitations in legal protection. Other Pakistani women of all economic and social classes face varying degrees of discriminatory and repressive behaviour, which not only reduce their life chances, but also make them vulnerable to HIV infection. However, the factors that marginalise people and render them vulnerable to HIV are quite visible like elsewhere in the region. Sex workers, both male and female, are widely available and the condom use is quite low. Nearly 70 per cent of the HIV transmission is through the sexual route.

Sexually transmitted infections (STIs): Personal awareness and knowledge of reproductive health issues is limited, and often erroneous, among the men and women of Pakistan due in part to the generally low levels of education, and also due to their limited access to effective reproductive health services. Men and women alike are often unaware of the differences between reproductive and sexual health and reproductive and sexual disease. When they do become aware of a possible sexual or reproductive problem, they often seek care from traditional healers (hakims) or from one of the many unregulated 'sex clinics' in the informal health sector. In addition, it is estimated that only 60 per cent of the country's population have access to the formal health care system and many (through personal preference or necessity) resort to the use of hakims, or traditional healers. It is not uncommon for clinics in villages to be operated by self-described 'doctors' who may actually have little or no formal medical training. This reliance upon unqualified practitioners may compound the risk of further infection due to their lack of knowledge and the possibility of inadequate infection control during their therapeutic procedures. Health care professionals generally believe, however, that the incidence of STIs in Pakistan may be increasing due to the relatively widespread presence of risk behaviours.

Injecting Drug Users (IDUs): IDUs are at a high risk of acquiring HIV and other blood borne infections because they often resort to unsafe practices such as needle and syringe sharing. Although smoking and inhalation ('chasing the dragon') are still the most frequent forms of drug abuse in Pakistan, injecting drug use is thought to be increasingly common, especially in the large urban areas of the country. In addition to the risks associated with needle and syringe sharing, infected injecting drug users can pose a risk to others through sexual transmission.

Men having sex with men: While there is little documentation about the extent to which men engage in sexual activity with other men in Pakistan, the limited evidence available suggests that such activity does occur throughout the country. Anecdotal evidence indicates that sexual activity between men occurs relatively frequently in boys' hostels and jails; additionally, research suggests that sex between men is often practiced among long distance truck drivers. Finally, there is a small but highly mobile population of transvestites, transsexuals and eunuchs known as the hijra, who are known to engage in unsafe sexual practices.

Mobility and migration: Can create conditions in which people become vulnerable to infection. It is commonplace in Pakistan for men to travel away from their homes to find work, either within the country or abroad. This separation from their spouses, families and communities can result in loneliness and isolation, and can lead migrants to engage in social and sexual practices that put them at risk of exposure to HIV. In addition, though there is virtually no documentation of the HIV/AIDS-related risks experienced by the large numbers of refugees in Pakistan, global experience suggests that this population may be highly vulnerable to HIV.

Sentinel Surveillance Report

Thirty-nine laboratories throughout the country conduct HIV testing. The quality of the testing centres has been described as varying from excellent to rather poor. The National Reference Laboratory in Islamabad is the only public health facility to do confirmatory testing. Factors associated with underreporting are:

— Scarcity of trained epidemiologists within the health system;
— Weakness of reporting system in general;
— Limited knowledge of case definition among health practitioners.

Though reliable seroprevalence survey data is limited, data from other types of surveys and sources suggest that HIV seroprevalence among the general population is still low in Pakistan. For instance, one blood bank in Sindh found that of over 32,122 samples taken from family donors for thalassemia patients screened in 1998 only 2 were HIV+. The results of the most recent (1995) cross sectional surveys of several population groups can be summarised as follow:

Pregnant women

— In Lahore, in a sample of 2000 women, 0.6 per cent were found to be HIV+
— In Karachi, in a sample of 2020 women, no cases were found
— In Faisalabad, in a sample of 900 women, no cases were found
— In Mirpur, in a sample of 295 women, no cases were found

TB patients (Patients with a new diagnosis of TB with pulmonary sputum positive or sputum negative with extrapulmonary TB):

— In Quetta , in a sample of 210 patients, 2.8 per cent were found to be HIV+

Long-distance truck drivers

— In Southern Pakistan, in a sample of 255 drivers, no cases were found.

Drug Users (Patients attending a major psychiatric centre, no information about mode of drug use indicated):

— In Lahore, in a sample of 310 patients, 11.5 per cent were found to be HIV+

— In Peshawar, in a sample of 237 patients, 3.7 per cent were found to be HIV+

STD Data

— There is currently no STD reporting system in Pakistan, and therefore information about STD prevalence is limited.

— Gonorrhea and syphilis are notifiable diseases in Pakistan.

— A 1995 study of STD clinic attendees found:

  — In Karachi, in a sample of 402 patients, 17.1 per cent were found to be positive for Syphilis and 2.9 per cent were found to be positive for Gonorrhea

  — In Lahore, in a sample size of 295 patients, 3.7 per cent were found to be PA+.

Poor availability of epidemiological data precludes proper assessment of the HIV situation in Pakistan. There has been some testing among antenatal clinic attendees in Pakistan since 1992. In 1995, no positive results were found in Faisalabad and Karachi. In Lahore, 0.6 per cent of women tested were positive. Between 1992 and 1999, there was no evidence of infection among women tested outside the major urban areas. In 1997, 0.2 per cent was found to be infected. In 1995, 0.2 per cent STD patients in Karachi and 4 per cent in Lahore were found to be positive. Testing among truck drivers in Karachi in 1995 showed no evidence. One study in 1996 found that 11 per cent of Injecting Drug Users in Lahore were positive. Cases have been reported from all four provinces, from the federally administered territories and also from Azad Jammu and Kashmir (AJK).

Figures	*Value*	*Year*
Estimated Number of HIV cases (Adults and children)	78,000	2001
Adults (15-49 years)	76,000	2001
Women (15-49)	16,000	2001
Women (15-49)	2200	2001
Estimated number of deaths due to AIDS	4500	2001
Estimated Number of AIDS orphans	25,000	2001

In 1997, the prevalence among sex workers in a red light area in Multan, a large city in Punjab province, was only one per cent. Among STD patients in Karachi, it was below one per cent in 1995. In Lahore, the capital of Punjab, it was four per cent. However, the factors that marginalise people and render them vulnerable to HIV are quite visible like elsewhere in the region. Sex workers, both male and female, are widely available and the condom use is quite low. Nearly 70 per cent of the HIV transmission is through the sexual route.

In 1988, shortly after the diagnosis of the first HIV/AIDS cases in the country, the Ministry of Health of the Government of Pakistan established the National AIDS Control Programme (NACP), based at Pakistan's National Institute of Health. The first government-funded programme plan for the NACP was developed and budgeted for a period of three years in 1990, and by 1994 the work of the NACP was expanded through the approval of a PC-1 for an increased financial commitment for the years 1994-97. By the end of June 1997, however, a sum of only about 15 per cent of the actual requirement had been made available to the NACP, and the duration of the original PC-1 was therefore extended up to 2003. Despite the Programme's inclusion in the Social Action Programme (designed to enhance government spending in the social sector) since 1997, and due to a myriad of issues, budgetary allocations have not matched the programme requirements. Despite these budgetary limitations, the NACP has played an important role in the creation of awareness about HIV/AIDS in Pakistan through an extensive general public awareness campaign. This effort has included the publication of educational materials, many different types of workshops and educational events, and an electronic media campaign.

In 1987, the Federal Committee on AIDS defined broad policy guidelines, which were, to a large extent, laboratory oriented. In 1994, the National Economic Council approved a broader National AIDS Prevention and Control Programme from 1994 to 1997. In 1994, the AIDS programme, along with three preventive health programmes was brought under the Social Action Programme (SAP), a Government initiative supported by the World Bank. SAP policy reform, targeted for 1997 to 2002, was adopted. HIV/AIDS is included in this phase too. The National AIDS Programme (NAP) has placed its initial emphasis on the development of laboratory services and surveillance. Later, high priority was given to the development of a programme management structure and strengthening of the NAP at federal and provincial levels.

The National Institute of Health (NIH) has been assigned to implement the NAP. The STD and AIDS programmes are grouped in a single unit. Provincial implementation units for AIDS control and safe blood use have been established in four provinces and two federally administered areas. A comprehensive awareness strategy has been implemented and 39 countrywide surveillance and diagnosis centres have been established. The mainstay of the AIDS Control Strategy in Pakistan is Prevention. The salient features of the strategy are:

— *Gross enhancement of resources:* The Government itself sponsors about 80 per cent of the total budget for AIDS Control in Pakistan.

— Decentralisation of HIV/AIDS Control Programme up to the provincial level through the development of Provincial implementation units in all the provinces of the country.

— *Development of a comprehensive HIV/AIDS awareness raising strategy:* This includes mass media campaign through electronic and print media. Besides, the NGOs are being continuously supported and NGO consortia on HIV/AIDS have been established in all the provincial headquarters. The campaign has paved the way to overcome the social and cultural barriers in raising general awareness regarding the sexual and reproductive health issues.

— *The national policy also includes strengthening of a national HIV/AIDS surveillance system:* The government has been providing logistic support for free HIV antibody testing in the public sector. The government is committed to institutionalise behavioural and serological surveillance through establishment of second-generation surveillance system.

— The public sector blood banks are supported for provision of free HIV and Hepatitis B screening since 1995 under the government initiative for promoting safe blood transfusions. The government is finalising the legislative framework for safety of blood.

— The National AIDS Control Programme serves as a resource centre to develop country-specific guidelines and protocols and for human resources development covering various aspects of HIV/AIDS including counselling, care, support, clinical management, STIs care, surveillance, and blood safety.

— *There is a clear focus on bio-social research:* Two national studies on 'Prevalence of STIs' and '2nd HIV Scro-prevalence' are presently being carried out. Pakistan is about to launch the second Knowledge Attitude and Behaviour Survey at the national level to determine the impact of media campaign. Simultaneously, an external evaluation of the national programme will also be carried out. All these studies will provide strong and evidence-based information for the planning of AIDS control activities in future.

— Government of Pakistan, in collaboration with UNAIDS and its co-sponsors has developed a 'Strategic Framework' for the next five years. This framework has identified nine priority areas which include: expanded response, vulnerable and high-risk groups, youth Surveillance and research, care and support, general awareness, blood and blood product safety, STIs and infection control.

Pakistan's Federal Ministry of Health initiated a National AIDS Prevention and Control Program (NACP) in 1987. In early 2001, NACP developed a National HIV/AIDS Strategic Framework to guide the activities of the HIV/AIDS stakeholders in Pakistan. This framework states nine priority areas including a coordinated, multi-sectoral response, reduction of 'risk' among high-risk groups, reduction of vulnerability among youth and improved quality of care for people living with HIV/AIDS.

Multisectoral responses and leadership: The national strategy has listed one of its priorities as being 'expanded response', which calls for effective and multisectoral partnerships at all levels. While conceding that political will and commitment against HIV/AIDS has been weak in the past, it advocates for support from the highest political levels. One of its 'priority area goals' includes a sustainable multisectoral response through organising sensitisation sessions for federal and provincial government officials. One of the potentially useful recommendations arising out of the strategy include the revitalisation of Pakistan's 'multisectoral Federal Committee on AIDS', which reportedly has PLWHA and NGO representation, besides that of provincial health ministries.

Advocacy: The strategy delineates the need for intensive advocacy with political leadership, international exchanges and the sharing of national and international 'best practice' experiences. It states that the weak response among policy makers in recognising HIV as 'a real threat to public health' is a major stumbling block. Advocacy with religious leaders and local communities to reduce stigma and discrimination finds mention. Several activities have been suggested, related to the production of IEC materials, mainstreaming HIV into existing mass organisation structures such as trade unions, peer education initiatives and facilitating sensitive media reporting. In spite of a few innovative activities, a wider focus on advocacy and policy dialogue is lacking, which would serve to interlink the various focus areas in an integrated manner.

Capacity development: There exists a list of blood safety and infection control mechanisms including guidelines on MTCT and surveillance strategies. Formalising referral systems, adapting VCT guidelines and appropriate usage of ARVs are also stressed. The document also states that there exist no guidelines for infection control.

Human Rights

Sex workers and MSM: The strategy lists 'high risk groups' as a separate priority area and this includes sex workers and MSM. It also suggests activities such as pilot peer education programmes and harm-reduction initiatives. Issues concerning sex workers' rights and MSM rights.

PLWHA: The Constitution of Pakistan prohibits the state from discriminating on grounds of sex, caste, race, religion, residence and place of birth in matters pertaining to access to public spaces and employment . If applied, this principle should also extend to include discrimination on the basis of HIV status in state run medical institutions. The priority areas as articulated in the national strategy includes increased knowledge and compliance with universal precautions within the health care setting, and improved quality of care for PLWHA, although the approach remains welfare based and lacks in a strong human rights component. Even though the inclusion of human rights groups for monitoring instances of stigma and discrimination faced by PLWHA is mentioned, actual implementation would need to be monitored.

Achievements

- Provincial Implementation Units for AIDS control and safe blood transfusion have been established in 4 provinces and 2 federally-administered areas.
- A comprehensive awareness-raising strategy has been developed and implemented through activities such as electronic and print media campaigns, telephone hot-lines, support to NGOs, district networking and imparting AIDS education to key influential persons.
- 39 countrywide surveillance and diagnosis centres have been established
- Broad policies for the essential screening of blood before transfusion have been adopted for interrupting transmission of infectious diseases such as AIDS.
- National guidelines on safety of blood transfusion and standard operation procedures (SOPs) have been prepared
- Public sector blood banks screen blood for HIV and hepatitis B virus
- More than 300 training workshops and meetings on different aspects of HIV/AIDS have been conducted since 1987
- In close collaboration with the Multi-donor Support Unit (MSU), the Social Action Programme (SAP) policy reform matrix and budget plans have been developed up to year 2002.

Support by Other Ministries

- In 1997, working closely with the NAP and sponsored by WHO, the Ministry of Labour and Manpower's

Directorate of Worker Education (DWE) implemented a set of 23 awareness-raising seminars for factory labourers throughout the country.

— The Ministry of Education has formulated a new National Education Policy, which includes HIV/AIDS education at the secondary level. This policy awaits approval by the National Assembly.

HIV/AIDS-Related Legislation/Policies

— HIV/AIDS was declared a notifiable disease in 1988.

— Foreigners living in Pakistan for longer than one year are subject to mandatory HIV testing.

— A federal legislation bill for mandatory testing of blood products used for transfusion is in the Senate for approval. Similar provincial bills have already been passed in Sindh and Punjab provinces.

— The National AIDS Programme has been included as part of the GOP Social Action Programme since 1994.

REFERENCES

South Asia HIV/AIDS Overview, The World Bank Reprot, 2002.

HIV/AIDS Surveillance Database, US Census Beuro, 2001.

5

Bangladesh: An Unfinished Data

The first patient with Acquired Immunodeficiency Syndrome (AIDS) was diagnosed in Bangladesh in 1989. Until 1999, ten AIDS cases and 126 persons with HIV infection. Currently available data show that HIV prevalence is still low. However, the paucity of data calls for a cautious appraisal. Indeed, many factors suggest that HIV may spread rapidly in the near future. These include high rates of sexually transmitted diseases and hepatitis B; significant number of commercial sex workers; evidence of high-risk behaviours; a large international and national migrant labour force; an essentially unscreened blood supply system derived mostly from professional blood donors, approximately 20 per cent of whom test positive for hepatitis B and syphilis; and rising injecting drug use.

The present HIV situation could, therefore, evolve rapidly into an impending and escalating epidemic. This window of opportunity of existing low prevalence should, therefore, not be missed to initiate primary preventive efforts. The national response has included establishment in 1985 of a National AIDS Committee (NAC), and Technical and Co-ordination Committees at central level and committees at various peripheral levels. A number of activities have been implemented by the NAC, the Ministry of Health and Family Welfare (MOHFW) as well as by the Directorate General Health Services (DGHS). A well-established NGO network carries out various HIV/AIDS related prevention and care interventions. However, in spite of a substantial amount of work already done, the level of response has been neither adequate nor satisfactory. The Government expression of commitment to AIDS prevention has to be translated into action at the ground level. The Government's Strategic Plan provides a framework for a national response to AIDS and defines Bangladesh's strategies and priorities for STD/AIDS prevention and care for the next five years (1997-2002) in line with National Policy. The plan builds on work already done and emphasises a multi-sectoral response to the AIDS problem to include enhancing the involvement of various Governmental Ministries, NGOs, the private sector and the community; and outlines programme management aspects including monitoring and evaluation. It also provides a guide for further planning and for the development of sector-specific work plans, which will follow.

The broad strategies and interventions included in the strategic plan take into consideration the present epidemiological situation and the likely future scenario. The priority strategies include:

— Establishing and keeping a NAP management team effective at central, district and upazila levels.

— Preventing transmission of HIV through expansion of interventions targeted among individuals with high risk behaviours including sex workers and their clients, truck drivers, injecting drug users, etc.; strengthening STD case management to include syndromic approach; increasing availability, accessibility and use of quality condoms; promoting responsible sexual behaviour of young people both in and out of school; information, education and communication (IEC) activities targeted at policy makers and the general population; enabling legislation and the use of the media, and above all creating an enabling environment for people in general and for those afflicted in specific which would include making information and care available to them.

— Improving a safe blood supply through promoting voluntary blood donation and banning professional blood donation;

— Rational use of blood/blood products and a thorough screening of donated blood for HIV and other pathogens;
— Provision of counselling and other support including expansion of voluntary testing facilities targeted at pregnant women or women contemplating pregnancy and breast feeding mothers;
— Provision of care and support systems including counselling services; implementing activities to include legal amendments to counter discrimination against people living with HIV/AIDS and vulnerable groups, towards improving community acceptance;
— Establishing HIV/AIDS and STD surveillance to determine present and future magnitude of the problem and to monitor HIV/AIDS and STD programmatic interventions and their effects;
— Strengthening capacity for diagnosis of STD/HIV/AIDS;
— Mobilising and supporting various Government, private and non-government sectors.

To guide activities related to these strategies and interventions, the National Aids Programme (NAC), recently approved a policy document on STD/HIV/AIDS, which has been accepted by the Government. Moreover, the Government is now fully committed to combat AIDS in Bangladesh and has accorded priority to STD/AIDS prevention and control. This is reflected by the Government commitment to establishing a NAP in the Directorate General of Health Services (DGHS) with full time staff to co-ordinate the overall national response and to provide technical and operational support to all sectors including NGOs and the private sector. Moreover, Government plans to ensure that all activities are planned and carried out within the framework of its strategic plan. The NAP will assist in coordinating HIV/AIDS prevention activities in various sectors, and facilitate decentralisation of activities to upazila and district levels. To do so, the NAP will establish links with upazila, district and division level AIDS committees and focal points in other relevant ministries and assist them in planning and implementing activities.

The NAP activities will be monitored by committees established at various levels, through regular reporting from peripheral to central level, and through field visits by the programme staff. External reviews of the NAP will occur every 2-3 years. To assess the progress made, indicators have been identified and targets set. To carry out various strategies and interventions included in the strategic plan, financial support would be needed. The Government of Bangladesh has committed required number of full-time staff to work at the national level and plans to set aside funds as a part of the 5-year plan. Additional resources would be mobilised from multilateral and bilateral agencies. The total budget requirements for the planning period (1997-2002). AIDS was first diagnosed in Bangladesh in 1989.

Since then, Bangladesh has 126 HIV infections and 10 AIDS cases, 6 of whom have died by 1999. The most common mode of HIV transmission in Bangladesh appears to be through unprotected heterosexual intercourse. Two children acquired infection through perinatal transmission. Unfortunately, the paucity of surveillance data means that HIV prevalence cannot be accurately determined. A protocol of HIV sentinel surveillance in Bangladesh was prepared in May 1994 with the assistance of WHO. Implementation was scheduled for 1995, which was delayed due to several administrative and financial constraints. However, First National Sentinel Surveillance was finally conducted in 1998-1999. The results showed that HIV zeropositive cases were present among the sub-populations practising high-risk behaviour such as injecting drug users (IDUs) (2.5 per cent), commercial sex workers (0.6 per cent), man having sex with man (0.2 per cent), and STD patients (0.1 per cent).

In spite of the low prevalence of HIV in the country, many factors suggest that HIV may spread rapidly in the near future. For example, studies have shown high rates of STD in various populations. In 1989, a syphilis rate of 56 per cent and 39 per cent were found among floating and institutional CSWs respectively. In 1997, 54 per cent of 980 CSWs gave a history of

Table 1
Estimated preliminary budget for the 5-year national AIDS programme

Broad Programme Area	*TK US$ ***	*Resource needs*					
		Year 1	*Year 2*	*Year 3*	*year 4*	*Year 5*	*Total*
Programme management							
Mobilising National	Tk.	1697.83	884.61	509.12	456.98	487.57	4036.11
International resources, Advocacy and Inter-sectoral	US$	4.04	2.11	1.21	1.09	1.16	9.61
Behaviour change intervention, IEC, NGO support and support to PLWHA	Tk.	1197.76	1279.95	1275.2	1042.75	1012.74	5808.4
	US$	2.85	3.05	3.04	2.48	2.41	13.83
STD Management	Tk.	472.56	573.54	518.34	427.54	162.86	2154.84
	US$	1.13	1.37	1.23	1.02	0.39	5.13
Condom promotion and harm reduction	Tk.	59.9	55.6	65.5	35.4	54.8	271.2
	US$	0.14	0.13	0.16	0.08	0.13	0.65

(Contd...)

Blood transfusion related activities	Tk.	421.08	426.31	319.72	52.68	28.19	1247.98
	US$	1.00	1.02	0.76	0.13	0.07	2.97
Care/counseling	Tk.	231	346.5	344.7	221	104.4	1247.6
	US$	0.55	0.83	0.82	0.53	0.25	2.97
STD/HIV/AIDS surveillance and Laboratory support	Tk.	98.46	126.46	133.21	97.29	72.46	527.88
	US$	0.23	0.30	0.32	0.23	0.17	1.26
Legislation	Tk.	56.36	61.73	52.65	50.73	51.43	272.9
	US$	0.13	0.15	0.13	0.12	0.12	0.65
Total	Tk.	4234.95	3754.7	3218.44	2384.37	1974.45	15566.91
	US$	10.08	8.94	7.66	5.68	4.70	37.06

Taka – Lakh
US$– Million

(Contd...)

present or past symptomatic STD. High levels of STDs amongst various other groups. As with many other Asian countries, condoms are not generally the preferred method of contraception. Furthermore, knowledge of condoms as a means to prevent STDs is very low. Moreover sex outside marriage might be more widespread than traditionally acknowledged. Documented practices include premarital, extramarital and male-to-male sex particularly among youth in Bangladesh. For example, some studies indicated a high percentage of youths with experience of sex before marriage and occurrences of induced abortions among women; sixty per cent of long distance truck drivers had sex with commercial sex workers about twice a month without knowledge of HIV/AIDS. Extramarital sex appears to exist in rural societies and in particular where husbands are absent for long periods. Important studies of the sex industry identify large numbers (100,000) of generally non-literate commercial sex workers (CSWs) whose customers represent all segments of society. Female CSWs have an average of 2-5 clients a day, making the number of clients about half a million men a day.

Bangladesh has large numbers of international and national migrant labourers, transport workers and uniformed personnel. These individuals spend extensive periods away from their families that contribute to getting involved in new and different types of sexual relationships. Transborder mobility is high. Bangladesh also hosts large communities of expatriate refugees while itself having nationals with refugee status in bordering countries. Available data from Client Monitoring System of Department of Narcotics Control and other research shows that prevalence of injecting drug use (IDU) is on the rise. Most IDUs in Bangladesh share needles. In some areas the professional injectors use one needle for many IDUs. There are estimated 20,000 IDUs mainly in Dhaka, Rajshahi, and other towns including bordering areas. Prevalence of STDs is quite high among drug users in general.

A high proportion of IDUs are clients of sex workers and many IDUs are married putting their family members at a higher risk of disease transmission. The First National Surveillance for HIV and syphilis among population practising high-risk behaviour showed highest zeropositivity for HIV among IDUs that was 2.5 per cent. The existing blood transfusion system also carries the danger of HIV transmission and therefore needs improvement. Problems include the need for approximately 200,000 units of blood, currently largely (70-75 per cent) provided by professional blood donors of whom approximately 20 per cent are positive for hepatitis B/syphilis. In addition to providing safe (screened) blood, the added risk of transmission caused by medical/surgical/dental procedures needs to be considered in the light of under-practised universal safety precautions.

Very little attention has so far been paid to the issue of mother to child transmission of HIV at any level. An effective awareness generation for all women, provision for counselling for pregnant women or those contemplating pregnancy, and breast feeding mothers, HIV testing facilities for consenting mothers, training of health personnel related to pregnancy and child birth and research on cost-effectiveness of anti-retroviral therapy are almost nonexistent. Bangladesh has many special contextual features which are relevant to HIV infection. These include widespread poverty, unequal access to health services, the often subordinate status of women, and low literacy and education levels. All combine to restricting knowledge in relation to health and negotiating power in matters of sex.

A multi-sectoral response and policy level support and commitment for empowerment of vulnerable groups to address the issues like stigma and discrimination are yet to be properly visualised. Research, specially operational research, in the field of HIV and AIDS is very limited in Bangladesh. Operational research is an essential component of effective implementation of any programme particularly those related to preventive actions and other cross cutting issues. The present HIV situation could evolve rapidly into an impending and escalating epidemic in the country with serious health and socio-economic consequences. The epidemic of AIDS could bring in future needs for major adjustments for individuals and their families, the health system, and within the community and society as a whole. An overburdened health care system both in terms of human and financial resources, disintegration of family structures, problems relating to increased poverty, numbers of orphans and abandoned children, and shortage of manpower in agriculture, industry and other sectors can be apprehended.

CONTROL ACTIVITIES

In October 1985, Government of Bangladesh (GOB) appointed a National AIDS Committee (NAC) with representation from different stakeholders. The NAC was defined as an advisory body with responsibility for major policy issues and strategies; co-operation and co-ordination of various sectors including NGOs; supervision of implementation of the programme and mobilisation of resources. A Technical Committee (TC) was formed, composed of experts from relevant fields to provide in-depth scientific, medical and technical advice to the NAC and the National AIDS Programme (NAP). By the end of 1990, a Co-ordination Committee (CC) came into being, constituted by key functionaries from institutions already engaged in HIV/AIDS related activities. Responsibilities were assigned to each member as part of a programme building effort. In 1987, GOB decided to start AIDS prevention activities with the technical and financial assistance of WHO Global Programme on AIDS (GPA).

In 1988, planned prevention activities began under a 'Short Term Plan' (STP) which focused on determining HIV/AIDS prevalence and in developing prevention and control measures, particularly in the health sector. During 1989, a 3-year 'Medium Term Plan' (MTP) was formulated and during the 90's, prevention activities were carried out with WHO support in areas of surveillance, laboratory diagnoses, and strengthening technical, financial, health education and management capabilities. Since 1996, UNDP has supported interventions in the country through the Bangladesh AIDS Prevention and

Control Programme. The Joint United Nations Programme on HIV/AIDS became operational in 1996 to work with Government, NGOs, the private sector, and donors to support the national response to HIV/AIDS. In appreciation of the complexity and gravity of the HIV/AIDS epidemic, the DGHS formed an 11 member 'Task Force' to initiate the process of policy formulation in 1995.

The national HIV/AIDS policy document was reviewed by a 19 member Core Group and examined by a multi-sectoral consensus workshop in which ten stakeholder groups participated in October 1996. The resulting final document was approved by the cabinet in 1997. The HPSP proposes restructuring of some components of the Health and Family Welfare wings towards unified service delivery. These factors need to be considered in formulating an effective management structure to deliver the health-related aspects of the NAP. At present, the government NAP management structure has been outlined in the policy document as follows: Programme activities are to be carried out by three main functionaries, i.e., the NAC, acting as an Advisory Body assisted by its Technical Committee, the MOHFW as the co-ordination body and the DGHS and other ministries, directorates and agencies as the Implementing Bodies.

The Technical committee (TC) is comprised of various specialists in fields relevant to the prevention and control of STD/AIDS. The composition is, therefore, continually reviewed to reflect needs as they arise. Important contributions of the TC include assisting the NAC to formulate programme frameworks; guiding programme personnel in the design, development and monitoring/reporting of their activities and review research protocols to be funded by the GOB. Programme management itself acts to maintain functional links effectively between the tripartite coalition. Terms of reference are being developed to clarify these links and to indicate how this committee can assist inter-ministerial functions.

Under the leadership of the Secretary, Ministry of Health and Family Welfare (MOHFW), the AIDS Information and

Awareness Campaign Committee (AI&ACC), comprising of representatives from several Ministries, WHO, donor agencies, media and NGOs, have conducted many activities in 1993 and 1994. Monthly meetings of the AI&ACC were initially held. Several Information, Education and Communication (IEC), materials have been produced and distributed by this committee. Other activities have included social mobilisation meetings, exhibitions and seminars in cities, towns and villages. Many media activities have focused on contexts in which people get involved in high-risk behaviours, as well as the public at large. However, means to redress religious and cultural sentiments, while still dispensing accurate information on means of transmission and methods for protection, need to be considered. Recent surveys indicate that literate and non-literate populations alike are generally mis- or uninformed about AIDS and are not empowered with sufficient information to protect themselves.

The availability of a quality condom at an affordable price is an essential component of any HIV/AIDS and STD control programme. At present, GOB provides 37 per cent of condoms while the remaining 63 per cent comes from the Social Marketing Company (SMC) funded by the USAID and the European Union. SMC has recently introduced a new brand with a clear message to link its use to prevent STDs and AIDS. A market has been established for this brand. The STD message should also be considered for all other condoms. For the first time SMC has also been allowed by the government to use TV for promoting condom for HIV. Condoms are also distributed free by many NGOs.

Approximately 200,000 units of blood are transfused in Bangladesh every year. Only a small percentage of these units are tested for HIV and other infections. With 70-75 per cent of the blood supply coming from professional blood donors of whom 20 per cent appear to have STDs, there appears to be a real danger for HIV reaching the general public through this route. In March 1997, a protocol for a safe blood transfusion service was submitted to the MOHFW by the Blood Transfusion

Technical Sub-Committee of the NAC. At present, a few laboratories have started to provide facilities to test for HIV in the country. Most are in the private sector. However, pre-, post- and follow-up counselling has yet to become an essential part of the process. As HIV/AIDS awareness increases, a rise in the demand for HIV testing is likely. To meet this demand, health facilities which offer voluntary counselling and testing would be required. As it stands now, MOHFW has embarked on establishing 97 blood transfusion centres in the country up to district level, some of which will in the private sector. These centres will screen blood for HIV, trepenoma, malaria, HBsAg and HCV.

NGOs have set up a STD/AIDS Network. It is broadly recognised that NGOs, given their potential for flexibility and interactive relations with community members, have much to offer towards prevention and behaviour change activities. Relevant to STD/HIV/AIDS, close collaboration between GOB and NGOs is currently being addressed. NGOs are being invited to support the MOHFW with delivery of the Essential Services Package (ESP); interventions for community behavioural change; training and providing standard guidelines for the programme. Non-Governmental Organisations have been carrying out the major part of HIV/AIDS prevention activities nationwide. From IEC, targeted interventions, to policy formulation, NGOs have been instrumental at all levels. Indeed, without NGO participation, Bangladesh would undoubtedly have been much further behind than it is at present. Furthermore, there is a network of media people (AIDS and Health Writers Group) and an AIDS and Legal Issues group (ALACAA). A successful consensus workshop was held (November 1995) to agree on the relative roles for GOB and NGOs towards HIV/AIDS prevention and control. In essence, NGOs have been given full support to complement GOB efforts and to take on activities which are beyond government's scope.

There are specific issues that AIDS brings to women. The disadvantaged and marginalised status of women in

Bangladesh deprives them of access to information and intervention programmes on AIDS as well as, most importantly, negotiating power in matters of sexuality. In response, a Women Wing (WW) of the NAC was set up to raise and plan for such issues within the NAC and the programme. In the NGO sector, women are taking part in programmes addressing the wider socio-developmental issues of women as well as providing information and behaviour change support to women. NGOs are also making a start to promote male responsibility in matters of sexuality and family planning. The role of the man as a dominant partner in sexual decision-making is often forgotten, perhaps because of the perceived difficulties. However, this is an area that obviously requires focused attention if a NAP is to be successful.

PROGRAMMING STRATEGIES FOR INTERVENTIONS

Priority Target Population

i) Sex workers and their clients
ii) Injecting drug users (IDUs) and their family members
iii) Male having sex with male (MSM)
iv) Migrant workers
v) Transport workers
vi) Young and adolescents.

Vulnerable Sub-population

The whole population structure can be categorised in to following sub-population according to vulnerability and according to the risk behaviour practiced:

High risk / core sub-population

i) *Sex workers*

Brothel based (recognised)

Street based

Hotel Based

Home Based (slum/community based)

ii) *Men who have sex with men*

Male sex workers and their clients

Non-commercial MSM

Hijras and their clients

Prisoners

iii) *Injecting drug users*

Injecting drug users

Sexual partners.

Bridge population

- Truckers (including helpers and cleaner)
- Other transport workers
- Young people
- Military/Uniformed forces
- Women in domestic work/workplace setting/garment workers
- Male Migrants
- International migrants
- Slum dwellers
- Working children
- Tribals

Low risk

- Secondary school boys and girls
- Men (15-45)
- Women (15-45).

Programme Priorities

In Bangladesh, HIV prevalence is still low with few diagnosed AIDS cases. Therefore, the priorities for the NAP under the strategic plan (1997-2002), are to prevent sexual transmission of HIV and reduce the vulnerability of populations with high-risk behaviours like injecting drug use. Immediate priorities, therefore, include implementing interventions targeted at individuals with high-risk behaviour, strengthening STD clinical management at the community level using syndromic approach, improving accessibility of various population groups to good quality condoms, and safe blood transfusion. In the area of care, priorities would include developing counselling services and taking measures to counter discrimination and stigmatisation of people with HIV/AIDS, towards enhancing their community acceptance. In addition, advocacy to mobilise political commitment, allocation of adequate resources, and multisectoral response and programme expansion to district and upazila levels will remain as priority areas. The following combinations of strategies and interventions are proposed:

Prevention of sexual transmission

The data available so far suggest that HIV transmission through sexual intercourse is likely to remain the predominant mode of spread. In addition, since HIV is essentially a sexually transmitted disease, most efforts and resources for prevention programme will focus on promoting changes in sexual behaviour which decrease HIV transmission. To that end issues of sexual negotiating power and conditions which render individuals' reproductive health dependent on others, need to be addressed. All interventions will keep the particular vulnerability of women in mind.

Expanding interventions targeted among populations engaged in high-risk behaviour such as sex workers and their clients, truck drivers, injecting drug users, groups practising male-to-male sex, professional blood donors and young people. Interventions will consist behaviour change communication (BCC) which will include peer education, community outreach programmes; enhancing availability of good quality condom, accessibility and its correct use particularly in risk situations; counselling, referral, networking and supportive mass media.

The role of community-based NGOs will be crucial. Other approaches would include education of young people both in and out of school.

Strengthening services for early STD diagnosis and management is now considered both relevant and important to Bangladesh because of the role these play in facilitating HIV transmission. The main thrust of the NAP will be to train primary health care workers (both government and NGO) at district and upazila levels on STD case management including the syndromic approach and supplemented by expansion of laboratory services where necessary and feasible, to provide effective treatment.

Resources are required to ensure regular drug supplies at all levels of health care services. Studies on STD treatment seeking behaviour, particularly among women, and to monitor antimicrobial susceptibility patterns will be conducted to support the NAP in policy and strategy formulation. Organised referral system, provision for counselling of the patients and their contacts, and training for all levels of service providers will be the other components of STD management.

At present, condoms are the only barrier method known to prevent HIV transmission during sexual intercourse with an infected partner. Quality condoms will be made available at affordable prices in as many outlets as is necessary for making the effort successful.

The NAP will complement the social marketing programme to ensure condom availability, accessibility, particularly in all situations of risk and to promote condoms for STD/HIV prevention. In future, when other devices become available programmes on those will also be taken up and will be made known to the population in general.

Other activities for the planned period include AIDS education in the work places and among general population using IEC approaches such as mass media and other traditional methods. Public opinion makers, lawmakers, law enforcers and policy personnel will be oriented in particular.

Prevention of transmission by injecting drug use (IDU)

In many countries, the HIV epidemic has been seeded within and amplified among injecting drug users, leading to spread in the general population. In Bangladesh, injecting drug use is on the increase, therefore, interventions targeted at injecting drug users and their partners are important.

i) Interventions for harm reduction should be a priority. Whatever harm reduction interventions are already operational needs to be consolidated and extended to increase coverage. Activities targeted at IDUs need to be consistent with an overall drug abuse prevention strategy.

ii) Harm reduction strategies should include both safer injecting and sexual behaviour. There should also be treatment provision for STDs and drug addiction itself. The latter is all the more necessary because many IDUs want to leave the habit and receive treatment. Linkages may be established with existing recovery programmes.

iii) Functional constraints need to be overcome through advocacy and cooperation with relevant agencies including law-enforcing agencies (Department of Narcotics Control, Police). This will in consequence help to reduce stigmatisation and harassment of IDUs, and create an enabling environment for harm reduction and recovery programmes.

iv) Intervention in IDU should encourage self-help and community support groups. Many interventional activities may be transferred to these groups like peer education, outreach, condom promotion and involvement in recovery programmes.

v) Adequate resource needs to be allocated for a sustainable programme. Arrangements for monitoring and evaluation need to be agreed between the Government and NGOs working in the field. Operational research specially in the areas of harm reduction component must be an integral part of the strategy, so that the implementing agencies get adequate feedback, training and capacity building are accentuated and there is a wider dissemination of the impact of the programme.

Prevention of transmission through blood and blood product

Theoretically, transmission of HIV through the transfusion of blood/blood products should be easily preventable. The cornerstone of a safe blood supply is voluntary, non-remunerative, regular donations from low-risk populations. However, the existing supply source (70-75 per cent) of professional blood donors and the lack of infrastructure for screening of donated blood at any level are areas of major concern. In order to promote safe blood transfusion, a systematic programme of action will be developed including:

i) Reorganisation of the existing blood transfusion services;

ii) Expansion of HIV screening facilities at all blood transfusion centres;

iii) Promotion of voluntary blood donation through education and motivation programmes to dependency on professional blood donation system;

iv) Acting upon national guidelines and on going in-service training of health care staff on rational use of blood and on promotion of universal precautions at the health care settings; and

v) Creating legislative provision to support safe blood transfusion strategies.

Prevention of mother to child transmission

The most effective way of preventing mother to child transmission of HIV infection is prevention of primary infection in mother and her sexual partner(s) through interventions. Given the current low level of HIV prevalence in Bangladesh, it is evident that screening during antenatal care will not be adequately sensitive and cost-effective. Therefore, priority for surveillance does not need any deviation from WHO/UNAIDS guidelines at this moment. However, following strategic initiatives should be taken during the plan period:

i) Provision should be kept for voluntary counselling and testing of pregnant women and women contemplating pregnancy, and specific protocol should be developed for the purpose, specially for vulnerable and bridge population, and piloted during the plan period. HIV counselling guidelines and related training materials should be reviewed to incorporate the issues of pregnancy and breastfeeding. All voluntary counselling and testing should be consistent with principles of human rights as outlined in the National Policy on HIV/AIDS and STD related issues.

ii) If HIV status of a pregnant woman is known, supportive counselling should be provided to her and to her family members. Counselling should include factual and accurate information about risks of disease transmission during pregnancy, childbirth and breastfeeding. Information on the benefits and risks of alternative feeding practices should also be made available.

iii) If a couple decides on termination of pregnancy, safe medical termination should be ensured. HIV-positive women and their families should be referred to available and easily accessible support facilities, if available.

iv) During all childbirth, a universal safe precaution should be ensured and added measures should be taken during delivery of a zeropositive woman. Training facilities should be created for FWVs and FWAs and suitable training modules should be developed for the purpose. Protocol for follow up of children of zeropositive mothers may be a part of the training module.

v) Provisions should be made for the use of short course of anti-retroviral treatment to prevent vertical transmission.

Enabling social environment

Working towards the goal of optimally humane and supportive care for people with HIV/AIDS will help reduce personal and social impact of the AIDS epidemic. This is specifically indicated for population with high-risk behaviour and general population with added vulnerability. As there are only a few AIDS cases diagnosed in the country, strengthening counselling services, to be delivered by health care workers and NGOs is an important priority. Moreover, as more HIV infected persons develop AIDS, care will become an ever-increasing part of efforts to limit the impact of the HIV epidemic. In due course, therefore, the need will arise to strengthen clinical management and provide care along the continuum from the institutional to the community and home level. Care will be taken to preserve confidentiality, avoid discrimination and help patients live normal productive lives. The broad strategies and interventions in this area, in order of priority would, therefore, include:

i) Further strengthening counselling and support services in relation to STD/AIDS diagnosis to provide psychosocial support including stress and anxiety reduction, and to enable individuals make informed decisions about HIV testing and plan for their future. Development and enhancing of capacity in both government and non-government sectors for the services like counselling and expansion of services and development of a well-organised referral system are essentially important requirement for the purpose. To be able to do so, male and female health care workers and NGOs will be trained in gender-specific counselling skills. Policy guidelines will be followed to ensure that no testing occurs without pre- and post-test counselling and informed consent.

ii) Expansion of other related services like referral system and service facilities for STD care, detoxification and recovery programmes for drug abusing population, income generation programmes for those who need economic rehabilitation will be part of the activities during the plan period.

iii) Minimising discrimination and stigmatisation of vulnerable populations as well as those with HIV/AIDS is essential for greater community acceptance as a prerequisite for providing community and home care. Community education and advocacy efforts to counter discrimination will be further strengthened. The media will be used to shape community acceptance of HIV infected people. National legislation will be examined and changed wherever necessary to support relevant behaviour change interventions, human rights, and voice some of the larger societal issues arising with national policy makers.

iv) HIV/AIDS care will be an integral part of the general health services. Health care workers will have the responsibility of providing care for people with HIV/AIDS and ensuring equitable access to care. Collaboration and coordination with various other health programmes such as tuberculosis, laboratory services, control of diarrhoeal and respiratory diseases etc., will be strengthened.

v) Support will be provided to NGOs and community groups in developing and conducting community-based supportive services. It should be emphasised that different population segments like adolescents and young people require different special approaches. Community mobilisation on positive health issues like voluntary blood donation and formation of functional self-help community organisations among people who need a supportive environment will support the above strategic efforts. Other activities would include training of health care workers on clinical management of STD and AIDS, strengthening of health care and laboratory systems, and logistic support like provision and promotion of condom, availability of drugs for STD treatment and required test kits. This all should be done for the practice of universal precautions at the health care setting and provision of required services for those who need them.

vi) Another important aspect of strategic plan for ensuring an enabling environment is information dissemination specially on the issues like adolescent sexual health, mother to child transmission etc.. Documentation of best practices will enhance the effectivity of any effort on information dissemination. It however needs continuous and consistent action research to keep the information up to date.

All such activities will be carried out in order of priority which may evolve with the epidemic in the future. It of course needs relevant guidelines for specific programme implementation so that a standard quality of activities and their outcome is maintained. This all should be done keeping in view the guidelines articulated in the national policy document.

Diagnostics, surveillance and research

Diagnostic facilities will be expanded and maintained. Such provision may be created in NGO and private sectors as well under the supervision and monitoring of the government and they will findings to the designated institution of the government [Institute of Epidemiology, Disease Control and Research (IEDCR)]. Research, specifically operational research on different programme implementation issues will be an important component of strategic plan. Operational research will be an integral part of any implementation effort from its inception. In this component special emphasis should be placed on the following:

i) Expansion of diagnostic services in a cost effective manner, monitoring of diagnostic centres and collection of diagnostic units by IEDCR.

ii) Periodic surveillance, both biological and behavioural, specially of high-risk population and general population with added vulnerability. Nationwide sample survey may be a long-term strategy.

iii) Priority areas of research may include study of knowledge, attitude and practice relevant to HIV transmission, condom use, utilisation of STD services, and also quality assurance of existing programmes and other similar issues.

iv) Development of Geographic Information System (GIS) to access to existing information and updates. Development of a Central Information Bank will be another priority.

v) Development of a system of dissemination of information to relevant agencies/organisations at regular periodic intervals or as and when necessary. Establishment of a clearinghouse may be an ultimate goal.

vi) Preparation of a directory of research organisations, specially those involved in health and other development issues.

Mobilisation of national and international efforts

Despite diagnosis of AIDS in Bangladesh twelve years ago, a comprehensive national response is yet to be mounted. To be effective, cooperation is needed across various levels of government, central, district and upazila; and between government and non-government including private sector, community and political leaders, as well as people affected by HIV and their families. Advocacy to encourage various key players to contribute to the programme effort is essential. Moreover, the national response needs to be built on existing local and national structures. The various committees established by government, the MOHFW and the DGHS have been very active in carrying out HIV prevention activities. However, these efforts must be planned and implemented in a coordinated manner. Focal points in other relevant ministries have also been identified. NGO networks for STD/AIDS and NGO focal points have been established who are enthusiastic and motivated to work on AIDS-related issues. Various UN agencies and donor organisations have also provided support in various areas. During the strategic plan period, it is proposed to:

i) Further advocate with policy makers at national, district and Upazila levels to mobilise and coordinate resources and to decentralise activities. Support will be provided to committees as well as to the programmes at each level for capacity building and responding to the AIDS epidemic.

ii) Continue to mobilise various sectors/partners to participate in AIDS prevention and control, and work with focal points in relevant ministries, and representative NGOs and the private sector to plan and implement AIDS prevention/education activities in phased manner.

iii) Provide training, material and logistical support to various organisations and sectors both within and outside the Government to include establishment of information resource centres, and advocate for policies as articulated in the national policy document.

iv) Involve all sectors in consensus building, as well as in the planning, management and evaluation of the NAP. A mechanism will be developed to facilitate dialogue between various partners on progress made and areas where support may be needed.

v) Mobilise international support for the multisectoral and comprehensive NAP.

vi) Monitor the spread and impact of AIDS epidemic in the country by setting up HIV/AIDS and STD surveillance by assessing the current HIV/AIDS situation and monitoring future trends by identifying the determinants of the epidemic spread and forecasting the future scenario. Surveillance data so obtained can then be used more effectively for advocacy as well as planning purposes.

Strategies of Interventions to Prevent HIV Transmission

Prevention of sexual transmission

i) HIV/AIDS education

ii) Counselling including partner notification and treatment.

iii) Develop voluntary counselling and testing at upazila/dist. and above

iv) Strengthen government, private and NGO services

v) Appropriate drugs and information, confidentiality, client friendly in dealing people coming for STD treatment

vi) Develop research

vii) Promote use of condoms for disease prevention

viii) Approval of BCC strategy and implementations.

Injecting drug use (IDU)

i) Peer education

ii) Targeted out reach

iii) Condom distribution

iv) Safe needle exchange

v) Substitution of injections with orals for harm reductions

vi) Health education and counselling

vii) Support groups

viii) Recovery programmes.

Prevention of transmission through blood / blood products

i) Establishment of safe blood transfusion services

ii) Expansion of screening services

iii) Encouraging voluntary blood donation.

iv) Capacity building

v) Safe blood transfusion regulation bill

vi) Decentralisation of hospital based services with provision of inclusion of VCT.

Prevention of mother to child transmission of HIV

i) Prevention of primary infection in mothers

ii) Reviewing and piloting issues and interventions for prevention

iii) Determination of priority of surveillance
iv) Expansion of voluntary testing and counselling facilities
v) Information dissemination on issues like HIV transmission and breast feeding
vi) Development of training protocol on care and follow up of HIV infected mothers and their children
vii) Adoption of safe universal precautions during all child birth
viii) Anti-retroviral treatment.

Supportive and enabling social environment and case management:

i) Creation of a supportive and enabling social environment
ii) Expansion and strengthening of STD services and merger of AIDS/HIV intervention into general health care services
iii) Community mobilisation and support for the formation of self help groups for people infected and affected by HIV
iv) Case management available whenever it is needed
v) Collaboration of different sectors
vi) Research and documentation of best practices.

Diagnostics, surveillance and research

i) Establishment and strengthening of existing diagnostic laboratories in a cost effective manner
ii) Conduct or support /commission continuous surveillance and periodic need based surveys
iii) Clinical research and documentation of best practices
iv) Operational research on programmes and their implementation.
v) Conduction of Geographical Information System and central data bank
vi) Development of directory of research organisations
viii) Dissemination of information.

Management mobilisation and co-ordination of national and international efforts:

i) Establishment and functioning of a programme management structure

ii) Mobilisation and coordination of national and international efforts to control HIV

iii) Secure high level and effective commitment

iv) Mobilisation and coordination of national and international efforts

v) Establishment of focal points and support plan actions of related organisations and ministries

vi) Mobilisation of international support and develop regional initiative

vii) Exchange of information.

TECHNICAL POLICY GUIDELINES

To address all social, ethical and personal issues related to HIV/ AIDS infection, the GOB has accepted policy guidelines for the NAP. These technical policy guidelines refer in particular to the following areas:

i) Surveillance of AIDS cases

ii) Testing guidelines

iii) Management of AIDS and HIV infection to include special groups, e.g. TB

iv) Behaviour change communication

v) Counselling of HIV/AIDS patients and confidentiality

vi) National blood transfusion services

vii) HIV/AIDS and women, men, children, adolescents, sex workers, IDUs, people staying away from their partners, prisoners, minority populations etc.

viii) Human rights issues

ix) HIV/AIDS education in and out of schools
x) Maternal and child health
xi) HIV/AIDS and the workplace
xii) Relationship of the NAP with other programme areas
xiii) Legal/ethical aspects
xiv) Social/behavioural/clinical research.

As programme needs continue to develop, National STD/AIDS policy will be consulted to ensure consistency. Moreover, in the area of political commitment, the GOB recognises that AIDS is a priority health and development problem in Bangladesh and expresses its commitment to allocate adequate financial and human resources to address effectively the growing HIV/AIDS problem. The Government would urge all its ministries, as well as the NGO and private sectors to get more actively involved in AIDS prevention and control in the country.

PROGRAMME MANAGEMENT

The National AIDS Committee (NAC) is a national advisory body that provides policy direction and advice on all matters related to HIV/AIDS. Chaired by the Honorable Health Minister, the NAC is composed of Ministers and Secretaries from all the related ministries and includes three Honourable Members of Parliament and leading experts from related fields. The terms of reference of the Committee and its membership is to be reviewed periodically to make it more effective and efficient. The Technical Committee (TC) is a technical arm of the NAC, comprised of leading experts from a variety of relevant fields including health, finance, media, education, legal issues, psychology, demography, religion, blood/blood products transfusion, academia, NGOs, human rights etc. Besides its policy and advisory capacity, the NAC will also promote, facilitate and co-ordinate a multisectoral response. The MOHFW acts as the coordinating and supreme Executive Body and the DGHS as the implementing body for health related activities.

Similarly, other ministries and their directorates, NGOs and the private sector will act as the implementing agencies for areas related to their respective fields. Each ministry will carry out AIDS prevention and control activities through their existing core administrative structures. A Coordination Committee consisting of line personnel relevant to various programme activities across different ministries will be formed to assist information and activity coordination. The NAP will provide technical and operational support to relevant ministries, NGOs and private sector in carrying out their specific activities.

An Executive Committee (EC) may be formed in the MOHFW with the Secretary as its Chairman to review implementation progress. A Focal Point (FP) at additional secretary level has been designated in the Ministry to coordinate the activities. Terms of reference have already been developed by GOB and EC membership agreed. The EC will review the recommendations of the NAC and generate executive orders for health-related implementation by the DGHS. The DGHS is to implement the health-related recommendations of the NAC under executive instructions of the EC through the AIDS Programme Manager via the individual Line Directors.

The Government has established an AIDS/STD programme under the DGHS. The AIDS/STD programme will be managed by a Programme Manager and supported by additional full-time staff including deputy and assistant programme managers (four each), and other staff members as appropriate under the leadership of Line Director.

Structure of NAP is given below. The Programme Manager will be responsible for the day-to-day implementation and coordination of HIV/AIDS and STD prevention and control activities while Line Director will be responsible for planning, mobilising as well as facilitating different actions by various actors/organisations. Functions of the NAP would be as follows:

i) Providing technical leadership and support
ii) Facilitating intersectoral collaboration and support, including various Government ministries, NGOs and the private sector.
iii) Mobilising donor support and resources
iv) Maintaining the inventory of technical and material resources including research
v) Ensuring capacity building through training and reorientation of all sectors
vi) Planning, monitoring and evaluation of the overall national programme
vii) Quality assurance
viii) Surveillance.

RESOURCES AND SUPPORT SYSTEMS

The implementation of the multisectoral activities in the plan will require mobilisation of additional national and international resources. This is likely to change as the programme needs become further defined. Mechanisms for fund-raising will be developed by each sector. The NAC and NAP will play a facilitatory role in coordinating these efforts. The following are possible sources/mechanisms of funding:

Local: Government may make financial and budgetary allocations to the various ministries and parent ministry/NAP for the prevention and control of HIV/AIDS; Community efforts and participation both in cash and kind will be encouraged including introduction of payment systems for certain services provided such as HIV testing keeping provision for the poor.

External support: External resources will still be required to complement Government and community efforts. Donor assistance will, therefore, be mobilised and channeled through one of the following:

i) Bilateral funding of the programme should be solicited by the Government. Such support will be administered by the Government to finance priority activities.

ii) Multilateral funds to be provided by UN agencies for support to various activities planned in collaboration with the NAP and according to the priorities in the described strategic plan.

iii) NGOs may raise funds and mobilise support directly from donor, Government and other sources for the implementation of AIDS related activities. The amount NGOs raise will have to be reflected along with activities in the Government plan and NAP should be informed by both donor and the concerned NGO about this.

The Government will facilitate or provide full time regular staff to work on the NAP and also provide office space, equipment and furniture etc. However, many programme staff as well as the focal points in various sectors, will need capacity building through training. The NAP will facilitate this training support as a crucial input for effective programme management at the central, district and upazila levels. Efforts to ensure sustainability of the NAP require high-level political commitment, full integration of the Programme, multisectoral participation and diverse national and international funding sources. Sustainability through cost sharing and cost recovery will also be considered keeping provision for poor who cannot afford alternative approaches towards the long-term management of the programme.

Management of National Fund

The NAP will be responsible for facilitating coordination of administrative procedures related to finances and for prompt implementation of activities. Given the current approved structure for the programme, the management of national resources for AIDS activities shall be the responsibility of the Secretary, Ministry of Health and Family Welfare.

PROGRAMME INDICATORS AND TARGETS

To evaluate the impact and effectiveness of the programme, targets and indicators have been identified. These include targets in the areas of prevention, care, as well as programme management. Process, output and impact indicators for each strategic area have been enlisted below. Additional specific short-term targets and indicators could also be built into the workplans for monitoring the implementation of NAP activities.

Prevention Indicators and Targets

Knowledge of preventive practices

— By 2001, 80 per cent of the population between 15-49 should be able to mention two ways of protection from HIV infection.

Condom availability

— By 2001, 150 million condoms will be available for distribution during the preceding 12 months.

— By 2001, all Upazila Health Complexes will have had 100 per cent uninterrupted supply of condoms in the preceding 12 months.

— By 2001, 80 per cent of the population between 15-49 years will be able to acquire a condom.

Reported condom use

— By 2001, 80 per cent of sex workers operating in brothels will the use of a condom during the most recent act of sexual intercourse.

— By year 2001, 60 per cent of truck drivers will to have used a condom during the most recent act of sexual intercourse if other than with wife.

— By year 2001, 60 per cent of migrant workers will having used a condom during the most recent act of sexual intercourse.

STD clinical management

— By 2001, 90 per cent of upazila will have at least one clinician trained in STD case management

— By 2001, 80 per cent of individuals presenting with STD in health facilities will have been assessed and treated according to national guidelines.

— All ANC clinics will assess and facilitate for clinical management for syphilis.

STD prevalence

— By 2001, the prevalence of urethritis among men aged 15-24 years will decrease by 50 per cent in relation to baseline data available.

— By 2001, the prevalence of positive serology for syphilis in ANC attendees aged 15-24 years will decrease by 50 per cent in relation to baseline values available.

HIV prevalence

— By 2001, HIV prevalence among women aged 15-24 years attending ANC will remain below 1 per cent.

— By 2001, HIV prevalence among CSWs will remain below 1 per cent.

— By 2001, HIV prevalence among IDUs will remain below 5 per cent.

Screening blood for transfusion

— By 2001, 97 blood centres will have developed blood testing for HIV, syphilis and HBsAg and HVC.

— 100 per cent of blood donated for transfusion will be routinely screened for HIV antibodies.

Care Indicators and Targets

Counselling services

— By 2001, 100 per cent district hospitals will have at least one staff member qualified as a counsellor.

— By 2002, 100 per cent of HIV infected persons will have received counselling by an adequately trained counsellor.

Clinical management of AIDS

— By 2001, 90 per cent of Upazilas will have at least one clinician trained in AIDS clinical management.

— By 2000, 90 per cent of AIDS patients in the district hospitals will receive clinical management according to national guidelines.

Programme Management-related Indicators and Targets

— By 2001, 100 per cent of brothels in the country will be participating in HIV/AIDS prevention activities.
— By 2001, 90 per cent of relevant ministries of Government will have initiated HIV/AIDS/STD prevention and control activities.
— By 2001, 80 per cent of NGOs involved in health related areas will have integrated AIDS/STD prevention and control activities into their on-going programmes.
— By 2001, 100 per cent of government, NGO and private concerns involved in AIDS/STD related interventions will be regularly sharing their activity with the NAP.

MONITORING

Programme Monitoring

Programme activities will be monitored by the AIDS committees established at central, district and upazila levels by quarterly from peripheral to the central levels, and through visits made by programme staff. The NAP programme activities carried out, deviation if any, from the planned programme and with regard to any specific support required. The NAP staff will regularly make visits to support various actors and to establish close collaborative relationships.Moreover, the programme will develop a management information system which will permit the tracking and sched-uling of activities so as to enable the NAP to monitor the imple-mentation of its work plan. At the same time, this system will provide for reporting on indicators and targets established and hence facilitate strategic planning.

Co-ordination

Establishment of linkages between various intervention levels including NGOs will facilitate more effective provision of programme support and will ensure better programme monitoring and improvement of programme design. This will promote active participation of the community in these activities.

Monitoring of the AIDS Epidemic

The progress of the epidemic in Bangladesh will be monitored by expanding and proper homing of the sentinel surveillance system for HIV. This will involve collecting baseline information and monitoring trends of HIV infection in specific population groups. Special studies to monitor gonococcal antimicrobial susceptibility will be carried out and data obtained on screening of donated blood will be monitored. STD prevalence data will also be collected and used for the monitoring of impact of HIV/AIDS prevention activities. The surveillance data will be disseminated to all relevant individual agencies and feedback provided to those collecting and sending data to the national programme.

Annual Reviews

Internal review of the national programme will be carried out annually by the programme staff themselves to take stock of achievements, constraints and methods for streamlining activities. Information on the progress being made to achieve specific targets defined in the workplans will be collected and analysed as appropriate. The annual report will contain a complete assessment of achievements and constraints in programme implementation, the lessons learnt, financial reporting and recommendations for future plans. The annual report will be shared and disseminated with NAC and development partners and other stakeholders as a basis for future planning.

External Programme Review

External programme reviews are necessary to more objectively evaluate the implementation of the NAP. External reviews will be carried out by a team composed of members outside of the national programme. These will include participation of the beneficiaries, various Government and non-government sectors, UNAIDS co-sponsors, UNAIDS and representatives of the donors. The external review should occur every 2-3 years. Participation of all interested parties will be encouraged so that repeated separate reviews by different donors can be avoided and discouraged. The review should look not only on the progress made in terms of activities but also assess achievements made on the targets already established in the strategic plan. It is expected that reviews will be undertaken under HPSP system.

REFERENCES

Government of Bangladesh, *Strategic Plan of the Natioinal AIDS Programmes of Bangladesh, 1997-2002*, July 2000.

South Asia HIV/AIDS Overview, The World Bank Reprot, 2002.

UNAIDS Report on the Global HIV/AIDS Epidemic, 2002.

WHO's Report on HIV/AIDS in Asia and the Pacific region, 2001.

6

HIV/AIDS: Impacts in Sri Lanka

In Sri Lanka, there are over 8,500 adults and children living with HIV, the virus that causes AIDS. Although the number of cases is still low compared to the total population, it is growing. International evidence indicates that there is only one thing that stands in the way of Sri Lanka as it is, and Sri Lanka with an AIDS epidemic: full understanding of the risks the country faces, and concerted, preventative action. The number of HIV/ AIDS cases in Sri Lanka is still low, but risky situations and behaviours that facilitate rapid spread of the infection, are widespread, making the country highly vulnerable to an HIV epidemic. Sri Lanka presently has a window of opportunity act vigorously to forestall a large-scale epidemic.

According to UNAIDS estimates, in Sri Lanka, the HIV infection rate among adults, between the ages of 15 and 49, is 0.07 per cent. Since 1986, only 405 cases have been officially reported. Under-reporting is due to a limited capacity for voluntary counselling and testing, and a prevailing stigma and fear of being identified or detected as HIV positive. While men outnumber women in the early phases of HIV epidemics, the number of women infected almost equals the number of men (the current ratio of HIV positive men to women is 1.4 to 1). This is largely due to women comprising the majority of emigrant labour to the Middle East who are required to be tested for HIV.

Although the overall HIV prevalence is low, extensive risk factors and behaviour patterns, which facilitate rapid spread of the infection, are widespread and make Sri Lanka highly vulnerable to an HIV/AIDS epidemic. These risk factors include:

i) *Low condom use*: Although research on sexual behaviours has been limited, a few studies conducted in the urban areas suggest low condom use among men. For example in 1997, only 4.7 per cent of men between the age of 15-49 in Matale and 9.6 per cent of men in Colombo reported ever having had used condoms, although about two thirds of them had heard about them. Among men who declared that they have had sex with casual partners during the last 12 months, only 26.3 per cent in Matale and 44.4 per cent in Colombo reported using a condom.

ii) *Commercial sex*: It is estimated that about 30,000 women/girls and 15,000 boys work in commercial sex. The risk of sexual spread among those engaged in sex work is heightened by low condom use and prevalence of STDs. In one study 45 per cent of female sex workers had experienced multiple STDs, and 70 per cent of male patients at STD clinics had reported frequenting sex workers. In addition, women and children in prostitution are considered most vulnerable to HIV infection, because they often lack the ability or power to negotiate condom use with clients or to seek STD treatment. They are often "hidden," creating a challenge for HIV prevention services to reach them.

iii) *Sexually Transmitted Diseases*: Every year, estimates of STD cases that are detected vary from about 60,000 to 200,000, of which only 10 per cent - 15 per cent are seen in the government clinics. This is a concern because STDs facilitate the spread of HIV infection and serve as indicators for low condom use and other high-risk sexual behaviours. Seventy per cent of male patients at STD clinics had reported frequenting sex workers, and 45 per cent of female sex workers had experienced multiple STDs.

iv) *High mobility*: Migration within Sri Lanka and to neighbouring countries such as India, where HIV prevalence is higher-is necessary for the economic survival of many households in both rural and urban areas. Thousands of women and men live away from their families as migrants abroad and as workers in the Free Trade Zones and plantations. Removal from traditional social structures, such as family and kin, has been shown to promote unsafe sexual practices, such as engaging in multiple sexual partners and in casual and commercial sex, as well as to increase vulnerability of women and girls to sexual abuse.

v) *Injecting Drug Use*: Sri Lanka has an estimated 30,000 drug users, of whom about 2 per cent inject drugs. Although there have been no reported cases of HIV thus far, this group is at high risk because of needle sharing. Drug users often experience difficulty accessing information and preventive and support services.

NATIONAL RESPONSE

In Sri Lanka, as in all the nations of Asia, policies to prevent the AIDS epidemic and to mitigate its impact must be at the centre of development policies and programmes. In 1992, the Government of Sri Lanka initiated HIV prevention and control efforts through the National STD Control Programme. The NSACP, managed by the Directorate of Health Services in the Ministry of Health, is implemented in collaboration with the provincial directors of health services, STD clinics, and the National Blood Transfusion Service.

Since its inception, the NSACP has made significant progress in improving STD services through refurbishment of clinics, meeting of staffing and equipment norms, and establishment of outreach camps. In addition, the programme has helped to ensure blood safety through screening of transfusions for HIV and upgrading of blood banks, and has increased knowledge of HIV/AIDS among the general population.

However, many challenges remain, such as increasing community-based preventive and care services for highly vulnerable populations and limited multi-sectoral involvement. Addressing these challenges, GOSL formulated the National Strategic Plan for 2001-2006, which indicates a significant shift in the national HIV prevention and control strategy.

Sri Lanka, with its deep historical commitment to human development, highly literate population, especially among women, and functioning health system, is in a strong position to confront and control the spread of HIV infection in the country.

The work of both local and international NGO's has been limited thus far, and their collaboration and coordination with the government needs to be expanded. In addition, NGO work remains largely uncoordinated and its programme coverage of high-risk groups is estimated to be less than 10 per cent.

Financial and technical assistance to the government and NGOs has been provided by multilateral and bilateral agencies, such as WHO, UN agencies, and JICA. Thus far, the World Bank has provided support of about $1 million every year to the STD/HIV programme through an ongoing investment project, the Health Services Project and is currently preparing to support a self-standing HIV/AIDS prevention project.

Government's priority concerns are:

i) Strengthen public health approach to HIV/AIDS prevention and control;

ii) Focus on behaviour change among population groups engaged in high risk behaviours, such as sex workers, and their clients, and transportation workers;

iii) Reach out to other vulnerable populations—such as youth, soldiers, police, internally displaced persons and workers in the Free Trade Zone and the plantation sector, and overseas migrants;

iv) Emphasise creating an enabling environment—policy, legal, social, and cultural—that will facilitate behaviour change and provision of support and care to those infected with and affected by HIV;

v) Call for a multi-sectoral response, involving other ministries, such as the police force and the military, and partnering with the private sector and civil society organisations, such as trade unions, religious groups, academic institutions, and NGOs.

Aware of the huge problems faced by neighbouring countries and those in Africa, Sri Lankan Non Government Organisations are not taking any chances and are using innovative methods to keep the spread of HIV under control. The prevalence of HIV/AIDS in Sri Lanka is lower than other nations in the region, such as Thailand, but infection rates are increasing across the country.

With assistance from the United Nations Children's Fund (UNICEF) a Sri Lankan NGO specialising in development communication, Worldview, has been using a new medium to communicate the prevention message in Sri Lanka — taxi drivers. These communicators are the three-wheel taxi drivers (TWTDs) who operate in the capital city of Colombo and the suburbs. They are also known as 'autos' or 'trishaws'.

It is estimated that there are over 60,000 three wheeler taxis in operation. Other taxis are limited in number and are relatively expensive. Therefore, TWTDs are the most popular mode of transport for all social classes, as well as for budget tourists. The nature of their profession means that TWTDs are close to the night life and commercial sex workers. Often they are 'contacts' or 'associates' for sex workers, which makes them an ideal medium to deliver safe sex and other HIV prevention messages to the community. To date, more than 6,000 TWTDs have been educated on the issues so far. Young people are more likely to catch HIV through unsafe sex than any other part of the community. With one third of the population under 24 years, UNICEF and its partners in the field face a significant challenge to stem the spread of HIV/AIDS.

School education programmes are an effective way to convey HIV/AIDs prevention messages to students. With 4.3

million children attending some 10,000 schools, teachers and peers play a crucial role in awareness of HIV/Aids prevention.

School health clubs, run by the students themselves, have the most direct impact in changing young people's sexual behaviour. By mobilising and participating in HIV prevention and health promotion activities in 11 districts, including rallies, marches, street dramas and other innovative communication activities, students have succeeded in promoting healthy lifestyles.

REFERENCES

Nishimizu, Mieko, "Sri Lanka, AIDS and Development", *The Daily Mirror*, Sri Lanka, October 29, 2002.

Sri Lanka, National STD/AIDS Control Sentinel Surveillance Reports, 1994, 1995, 1996, National AIDS Prevention and Control Programme, Ministry of Health, Sri Lanka.

7

Nepal's Strategical Analysis of AIDS Control

In the Human Development Report 2001, Nepal features among the economically poorest countries in the world. Nepal's social indicators remain well below the average for the South Asia region: more than 40 per cent of the Nepali population live below the national poverty line, nearly half of all children below 5 years are underweight and nearly 60 per cent of all adults are unable to read or write. Additionally, women have traditionally a lower status than men and gender inequality is deeply rooted.

Nepal is one of the few countries worldwide in which men live longer than women. More boys than girls receive any form of education, women generally work longer hours than men, and men have better access to services, including health. The pressure of population growth on scarce and fragile land means that the benefits of better education or irrigation are often outweighed by more fragmented land and reduced availability of forest products upon which most of the rural population depends for all or part of its livelihood. In Nepal, the topography, environmental degradation, poverty and economic migration are all linked and they combine with other factors to increase vulnerability to HIV.

Following are the epidemiological factors:

i) Predominant mode of transmission is sexual contact, presumably mainly heterosexual

ii) Limited information available about homosexual/bisexual transmission
iii) Highest rates of HIV have been identified in injecting drug users (IDUs)
iv) Data indicates that risk behaviours are widespread among sex Workers (SWs), their clients, injecting drug users, labour migrants and youth/young people.
v) Current estimated HIV infection rate — 0.5 per cent of the adult population between the ages of 15 - 49.
vi) There is evidence of an explosive increase in the number of infections since 1996
vii) Increasing levels of Sexually Transmitted Diseases (STDs) reported.

Male / female ratio

— Approximately 3:1 (NCASC, 2001)

*Geographic distribut*ion

— Highest prevalence rates found in the Central Region.
— Rural /urban ratio to be determined
— HIV infection has been noted in all regions of the country, although HIV infection appears to be concentrated in urbanised areas and districts with high labour migration.

Table 1
The HIV / AIDS Epidemiological Situation in Nepal

	Data	Date
Reported HIV cases	2392	June 2002
Reported AIDS cases	606	June 2002
Estimated number of adults & children living with HIV/AIDS	60,018	End 2002
Estimated adult and child mortality due to HIV/AIDS	2,958	End 2002
HIV prevalence		
IDUs	68 %	2002
SWs	17.3%	2000
STI patients	0.7-6.6	2000
Blood donors	0.28-0.48	2000
ANC	0.2%	2000

The first cases of AIDS were reported in Nepal in 1988. Surveillance data is scarce in Nepal. However, limited data indicate that HIV prevalence is currently around 0.5 per cent in the general population. As of June 2002, the Ministry of Health (MoH) has reported 606 cases of AIDS and 2,392 HIV infections. Given the existing medical and public health infrastructure in Nepal and the lack of continuity in national HIV/AIDS surveillance systems, it is very likely that the actual number of cases is many times higher. UNAIDS/WHO estimate for 2002 around 60,018 people living with HIV/AIDS, and 2958 AIDS related deaths in that year alone.

However, the currently low prevalence among the general population masks an increasing prevalence in several groups: SWs in Kathmandu 17.3 per cent, IDUs 40.4 per cent nationwide, and 68 per cent in the Kathmandu Valley. It is now evident that Nepal has entered a "concentrated epidemic", i.e. the HIV/AIDS prevalence consistently exceeds 5 per cent in one or more subgroups.

Among all IDUs in Nepal (estimated number 30,000), approximately 40 per cent are HIV positive, and among IDUs in Kathmandu (estimated 10,000-15,000) the rate has increased to around 70 per cent. In addition, a survey among 300 SWs in Kathmandu revealed that 15 women had also injected drugs, representing 5 per cent of the total sample. Of these 15 women, 11 were found to be HIV positive.

A survey in Kathmandu in 2000 revealed that 17.3 per cent of SWs were HIV-positive up from 2.7 per cent in 1996. It is estimated that as many as 70 per cent of SWs returning from India are HIV-positive. There are no national statistics for prevalence among SWs, but the proportion is high and no doubt growing.

Estimates of the number of Nepali men working in India are around 1 million and above. Migration to India will undoubtedly continue to increase in coming years. Many of these men are contracting HIV/AIDS in India and bringing it back to their wives in Nepal. A recent survey of men returning from Mumbai to Nepal revealed an HIV infection rate of 10 per cent.

Most of the 60,000 people living with HIV/AIDS (PLWHA) do not know they are infected and many of them may be engaging in unsafe sexual practices. Pervasive stigma and discrimination will prevent these people and others in the high-risk groups from practising safe sex, undergoing testing, and if they know they are infected from seeking treatment and care.

POTENTIAL FOR HIV PREVALENCE

Behavioural and seroprevalence data indicate the high potential for a generalised epidemic in Nepal. In the absence of effective interventions, even a "low to moderate growth scenario" would make AIDS the leading cause of death in the 15-49 year old population over the coming years. For Nepal this would mean that around 100,000-200,000 young adults will become infected and that overall 10,000-15,000 annual AIDS cases and deaths may be expected.

For Nepal, a generalised epidemic with high mortality in the productive age group would start a "vicious circle". The impact of HIV/AIDS would increase poverty and vulnerability. This increased vulnerability would lead to more HIV infections and a higher impact. Besides the negative impact on socioeconomic development and the loss of productive life, the burden of disease would change dramatically over the next 10 years and would put further stress on the health sector and local communities.

Sexually Transmitted Diseases

STDs also form a significant part of the epidemic. It is estimated that 200,000 episodes of STDs occur annually in Nepal. The STD prevalence rate in women is approximately 4.7 per cent ranging from 2.7 per cent - 5.4 per cent. Access to STD services is still very poor, especially for women. In addition, the use of condoms for effective infection prevention is not yet commonly known or accepted. Condoms contributed to only 1.1 per cent of the total contraceptive prevalence rate. At present other methods of contraception are emphasised, which leave women vulnerable to infection and force them to negotiate condom use for infection prevention.

In 1988, HMG/Nepal launched the first National AIDS Prevention and Control Programme. This programme, known as the Short-Term Plan for AIDS Prevention and Control, formed the basis for the First Medium Term Plan 1990-92. This programme was externally reviewed in December 1992 and on the basis of the recommendations made during the review, the Second Medium Term Plan for AIDS Prevention and Control in Nepal was formulated covering the years 1993-97.

In 1993, HMG/Nepal accepted the need for multi-sectoral involvement in AIDS and STD control and different focal points were appointed in various sectoral ministries. However, due to frequent political changes neither the National AIDS Coordination Committee nor the multi-sectoral coordination and cooperation has been fully functional.

In 1995, HMG/Nepal adopted a national policy for AIDS prevention, with 12 key policy statements which includes: priority to HIV/AIDS and STD prevention programmes; the need for a multi-sectoral and decentralised response; the acknowledgment of NGO implemented programmes, coordination; evaluation, services for people living with HIV/ AIDS; a nondiscriminatory approach, confidentiality for test results; and blood safety.

The National Centre for AIDS and STD Control (NCASC) was formed within the department of Health for the implementation of the AIDS prevention programme. Policy guidance for the NCASC comes from the National AIDS Coordination committee, a multi-sectoral body with participation from public and private sectors.

Based on the National Policy, a "Strategic Plan for HIV and AIDS in Nepal", covering 1997 to 2001 was developed and adopted. It tried to operationalise the national policy and to define key activities for each policy objective. Although the strategic plan contained a number of activities aimed at prevention of a fast spread of the epidemic, only few of them were actually implemented.

The strategic plan sought to broaden the response to other sectors beyond the health ministry and to integrate HIV/AIDS concerns within these sectors. Factors relating to mobility of populations, urbanisation, heavy labour migration to areas where huge infrastructure programmes are being undertaken, the open border between Nepal and India and poverty have been recognised as casual factors for the spread of the infection in the country.

Recently Nepal established a "National AIDS Council" chaired by the Prime Minister. The Council with representation from government, non-governmental organisations, private sector and civil society will take the lead in policy making and will advocate for multi-sectoral participation in the fight against HIV/AIDS in Nepal.

Strategic Plan in Nepal

There have been a number of important changes since the development of the "Strategic Plan for HIV and AIDS in Nepal 1997-2001":

i) The epidemiological situation has dramatically changed between 1997 and 2001;

ii) Nepal has committed itself both to the Millennium Declaration and its Millennium Development Goals and to the time-bound targets spelled out in the Declaration of Commitment at the United Nations General Assembly Special Session on HIV/AIDS in July 2001; and

iii) Nepal's Tenth Five-Year Development Plan has identified HIV/AIDS as a cross cutting issue affecting national development.

This new National Strategy should guide the translation of these commitments into reality and to finally halt and reverse the spread of the epidemic in Nepal.

The strategy development process was designed to be highly participatory and was undertaken in the following three stages:

Situational analysis

To provide a better understanding of the HIV situation in Nepal, the NCASC commissioned a Situation Analysis as a first step in the strategic planning process. Fieldwork for the Situation Analysis started in late 2000 with a report being published in December 2000. The Situation Analysis team performed a literature review, group discussions, and field visits. Those involved included government, external development partners, INGO/NGOs and members of vulnerable groups such as SWs, IDUs and PLWHA.

Response analysis

The response analysis highlighted the weak nature of the institutional response. For example, a number of ministries of HMG/N had some involvement in HIV/AIDS, but only a minority had integrated HIV/AIDS into their plans and budgets. The major burden for dealing with a multi-sectoral response to the epidemic has been left to the Ministry of Health which itself lacked the capacity to mount a response on the scale required.

A number of non-governmental organisations were identified who were actively engaged in responding to HIV. While some of their work appears to be highly effective, its coverage is insufficient to control the epidemic. Much of it is related to awareness raising which by itself is not enough to change behaviour, especially in the most vulnerable groups such as SWs, their clients and IDUs. In addition, current resources and institutional arrangements are inadequate to provide appropriate care and support to those infected and affected by HIV/AIDS. IDUs, SWs, their clients, and mobile populations were identified as vulnerable to HIV/AIDS not only because of their behaviour, but also because of lack of social and legal protection.

Development of the national strategy

A five member-working group, chaired by the director of NCASC was formed in December 2001 to facilitate the strategic planning process. In order to include all major stakeholders in the process, four theme groups were established covering the following priority areas identified by the situation and response analysis.

i) vulnerable groups
ii) young people
iii) care and support
iv) epidemiology and research.

A fifty group, composed of government official and external development partners looked at the management issues of an expanded response. These groups met between three and five times during February and April 2002 to develop, review and revise draft strategies. Participation in these groups was form all sectors, including people living with HIV/AIDS. Updated drafts of the strategy components were also posted on the internet and a special e-mail account was established for comment and suggestions from people who could not participate in the thematic meetings.

NEPAL'S HIV/AIDS STRATEGY

The overall objective of Nepal's strategy for HIV/AIDS is to contain the HIV/AIDS epidemic in Nepal. The vision of the

National Strategy is to expand the number of partners involved in the national response and to increase the effectiveness of the response. It will do this by focusing on activities within priority areas thereby optimising prevention and reducing the social impact of HIV/AIDS in the most cost-effective manner.

The strategy emphasises prevention as the mainstay for an effective response. It also highlights the need for care and support for people infected and affected by HIV/AIDS. This is not only important in it's own right, but it is also an important contribution to effective prevention. Considering the dynamic nature of the HIV/AIDS epidemic, the strategy acknowledges the importance of accurately tracking the epidemic and monitoring the effectiveness of interventions.

Nepal's "National HIV/AIDS Strategy 2002-2006" has been designed to guide the expanded response to the HIV/AIDS epidemic in Nepal. An expanded response requires the commitment of all sectors, not just health, both within and outside government, and the coordinated support of external development partners. This strategy will promote and facilitate the coordination of their involvement.

HMG/N Ministries should use the National Strategy to develop and integrate relevant elements of this document into their respective sectoral plans and policies.

Local authorities should use the strategy as a basis for developing their own strategic and operational plans according to their own needs. This document also aims to guide private and social sector organisations and external development partners in defining their support and contribution to an expanded response.

As this National Strategy describes the national priorities for the HIV/AIDS response, it should form the basis for future allocations of human, material and financial resources. The National Strategy is not meant to be a document purely for the government but needs to be equally owned by all stakeholders involved in the fight against HIV/AIDS in Nepal. Although this strategy will remain in place for five years it will be reviewed regularly and, if needed, adapted accordingly.

The HIV/AIDS epidemic has brought about challenges that are too diverse and complex to be tackled by government or by NGOs alone. It raises socioeconomic, legal, ethical and human rights issues that all need to be adequately addressed if the fight against the epidemic is to be successful. Partnership and involvement of all relevant sectors and a wide range of agencies and individuals including those directly affected by the epidemic are essential to any attempt to stop the spread of HIV/AIDS.

Nepal has been a signatory to a number of international declarations — the most recent being the UNGASS Declaration on HIV/AIDS agreed to in June 2001. In addition, Nepal has been a party to other key international agreements such as the "Melbourne Manifesto" emanating from the Sixth International Congress on AIDS in Asia and the Pacific in October 2001.

Further, Nepal has implicitly adopted the "Greater Involvement of People Living with AIDS Principle (GIPA)" through its participation and approval of the UNGASS and Melbourne documents and other international agreements. Thus, at the international level, Nepal has adopted a sound fundamental set of general guidelines and principles, which should underpin the national strategy. These guidelines and principles include:

i) *Multi-sectoral engagement*: As the epidemic is complex, affects all parts of society, involves individual, institutional and social behaviour, and far transcends the health sector, effective national responses must be multi-sectoral in spirit and structure.

ii) *Broad political commitment*: As the UNGASS Declaration states, "Leadership by governments in combating HIV/AIDS is essential and their efforts should be complemented by the full and active participation of civil society, the business community, and the private sector. Leadership involves personal commitment and concrete actions."

iii) *Civil society involvement*: As sub-components of a multi-sectoral approach and political commitment, the involvement of civil society is nevertheless worthy of highlighting as a central principle in the response. Without meaningful involvement of those groups representing all segments of society, the response will be inadequate. In particular, groups representing PLWHA need to be involved not only as meaningful participants in policy and programme discussions, but also actively involved in the organisations and agencies that implement programmes. The GIPA principle is a critical element.

iii) *Stigma reduction*: The adverse impacts of stigma and discrimination are being increasingly recognised as key barriers to combating the epidemic. Commitment to reducing stigma is therefore a central guideline and principle in all-international agreements.

iv) *Prevention to care continuum*: A keystone to the international response is recognition and adoption of programmes that address the epidemic at all stages from prevention to care, support and treatment. To wit: "acknowledging that prevention of HIV infection must be the mainstay of the national, regional and international response to the epidemic; and that prevention, care, support and treatment for those infected and affected by HIV/AIDS are mutually reinforcing elements of an effective response and must be integrated in a comprehensive approach to combat the epidemic" (UNGASS). Specifically, UNGASS emphasises "...that care, support, and treatment can contribute to effective prevention through increased acceptance of voluntary and confidential counselling and testing and by keeping PLWHA and vulnerable groups in close contact with health-care systems and facilitating their access to information, counselling, and preventive supplies."

v) *Human rights based approaches*: All international declarations reference the absolute need to take strong human rights approaches for combating the HIV/AIDS epidemic. The reasons for this are well documented and related to fundamental rights such as access to health care, information, and gender equity. In addition, human rights approaches have powerful programmatic effects as they reduce vulnerability to HIV/AIDS and also help prevent stigma and discrimination against people living with or at risk of HIV/AIDS.

Based on international commitments and principles, and on the findings of the situation and response analysis in Nepal, the following are the guiding principles for the design of HIV prevention and care strategies and interventions in Nepal over the next five years:

i) HIV/AIDS is more than a public health priority. It is a complex, multifaceted problem affecting all aspects of society.

ii) Multi-sectoral and interdisciplinary involvement is essential for building an adequate response to the HIV epidemic.

iii) The primary focus of the strategy will be on prevention.

iv) The response to HIV/AIDS will be rights based with a specific focus on the rights of people infected and affected by HIV/AIDS, in particular the right to confidentiality.

v) Resources allocated must take into consideration defined priorities based on the vulnerability of various affected groups and communities.

vi) People and communities must be empowered to protect themselves against HIV infection within a supportive environment.

vii) Equal access to basic care and services must be guaranteed for all persons infected and affected by HIV/AIDS.

viii) Gender considerations will be central to the development of programmes and interventions.

ix) Universal precautions must be well known and applied to prevent the possibility of HIV transmission through medical interventions and to prevent discrimination.

x) HIV testing must be voluntary with guaranteed confidentiality and adequate pre-and post-test counselling both in the public and private sectors.

xi) The participation of "target groups" in the design and implementation of programmes and projects is essential.

xii) Emphasis must be on involvement of people living with HIV/AIDS in the design and implementation of policies, strategies, programmes and projects.

The priority areas identified in the situation and response analysis that are addressed in the national HIV/AIDS strategy are:

i) Prevention of STIs and HIV infection among vulnerable groups.

ii) Prevention of new infections among young people.

iii) Ensuring care and support services are available and accessible for all people infected and affected by HIV/AIDS

iv) Expansion of a monitoring and evaluation frame through evidence based effective surveillance and research.

v) Establishment of an effective and efficient management system for an expanded response.

This strategy defines vulnerable groups as those whose lifestyles, social or professional context and behaviour make them most vulnerable to HIV/AIDS.

Although a number of groups and communities in Nepal have to be considered as "vulnerable", the groups identified as a possible nucleus for a generalised epidemic are SWs and their clients; injecting drug users; mobile populations especially labour migrants to India; men who have sex with men; and prisoners because of their extreme conditions.

The dynamics of the epidemic follow a predictable pattern — a rapid increase in the most vulnerable groups (e.g. SWs and IDUs); then a spread via "bridge populations" (e.g. clients of SW) into the general population. Therefore the top priority to prevent a generalisation of the epidemic in Nepal is to address the needs of the most vulnerable groups.

In the past interventions have been limited in terms of coverage, they also had to deal with an unsupportive environment and they did not sufficiently include members of vulnerable groups in the programming cycle. Members of most vulnerable groups are also marginalised within society and often do not enjoy their basic human rights. This strategy recognises the need to empower these groups so that they are able to protect themselves from HIV infection. To prevent STIs and HIV infections among SWs and their clients, injecting drug users, mobile populations — especially labour migrants to India, men who have sex with men and prisoners.

Sex Workers (SWs) and their Clients

Due to their highly marginalised status in society, SWs have little access to accurate information about reproductive health and STIs. Cultural, economic and social constraints limit their access to legal protection and to medical services. A survey by Family Health International in 1999 among SWs 4 and truckers along the high way routes in the Terai showed that 75 per cent of the truckers had sex with a sex worker and that only 70 per cent of the truckers had used a condom in the last sexual encounter.

The survey showed that the STD prevalence among the truckers was 10.2 per cent and the HIV prevalence was 1.5 per cent. As regards SWs, 69 per cent of clients were truckers and 51 per cent migrant workers. Only 40 per cent of clients had used a condom in the last sexual encounter. Overall, HIV prevalence among SWs was 4 per cent. Of those SWs who had recently worked in Mumbai it was up to 50 per cent.

A survey in Kathmandu in 2000 revealed that 17 per cent of SWs were HIV-positive — up from 2.7 per cent in 1997. It is estimated that 70 per cent of SWs returning from India are HIV-positive. There are no overall national statistics for prevalence among SWs but it is likely to be high and growing.

Most SWs experience increased vulnerability to HIV/AIDS due to a low level of education, which restricts access to information and health care services. They have little control over the risk in sexual encounters because the client often determines whether or not to use a condom. Moreover violence against SW is common.

Injecting Drug Users (IDUs)

Nepal was the first developing country in which an NGO established a "harm reduction" programme with needle exchange for IDUs and was until recently considered as an example of how early interventions could prevent the spread of HIV/AIDS in this community. Unfortunately, this perception proved to be misplaced.

Due to the limited coverage of interventions, HIV spread undetected among IDUs and a rapid assessment in 1999 5 showed an HIV prevalence among injecting drug users nationwide of 40 per cent and 68 per cent in the Kathmandu Valley. Behavioural research among IDUs in Nepal clearly indicates that needle sharing, the major risk factor for HIV, is common.

Although IDUs constitute the population subgroup in which HIV threatened to rise most rapidly neither governmental nor non-governmental capacity and policy were positioned to mount an effective response.

IDUs in Nepal are threatened not only by their behavioural risks but also by a societal response, which ostracises drug use and uses a predominantly punitive model coupled with limited drug treatment facilities. HIV and STI prevention services for IDU are often of questionable quality mainly because they are not designed with the needs of the end-user in mind. These limitations signal an ominous trend of increasing HIV prevalence among this highly marginalised group.

The main thrust of the strategy is therefore to establish an environment conducive to a rapid scaling-up of harm reduction interventions and to build the capacity needed to do so. The harm reduction approach gives drug users options to reduce their risk at various levels and focuses on supportive rather than punitive strategies. The strategy recognises that while stopping drug use is often the ideal goal, several intermediate goals such as safer injection techniques and drug treatment have to be implemented in order to stop HIV transmission among IDUs.

Mobile Population

"Mobility" has complex causes, ranging from economic and/or political reasons to "forced" displacement. Each of these mobile groups and their respective families are vulnerable to HIV/AIDS/STI in different ways. The aim of this strategy is to address the more behaviour related factors of HIV/AIDS/STI vulnerability, but at the same time to advocate for a holistic approach to address the broader determinants of HIV/AIDS/STI vulnerability among mobile populations. Economic migration, both internal and external is not a new phenomenon in Nepal.

Estimates range from 1.5 to 2 million Nepali nationals who work outside the country, 1 million are estimated to be in different parts of India alone. Although information is limited about the behaviour of labour migrants in their respective host countries, the assumption is that during their long absence from their families a considerable number of them become clients of SWs. Recent studies among labour migrants revealed

HIV sero-prevalence rates of between 2-10 per cent for migrants returning from Mumbai/India.

Estimates of women trafficked to India range from between 150,000 - 200,000. Conflict triggered migration from rural areas in Nepal to urban centres is not exactly known but is thought to be considerable.

Nepal's response cannot address the needs of mobile populations whilst they are outside the country. Research and targeted interventions on HIV/AIDS/STI aimed at this population whilst they are in Nepal is a priority considering the large numbers and the high potential for a spread of HIV/AIDS/STI to the general population through their partners.

Only recently have small surveys reported that sex between men seems to be relatively common in Nepal, particularly within Kathmandu. In this marginalised community many of the men engaged in casual sex with other men neither have the knowledge nor practice safe sexual behaviour when having sex with their male partners. Furthermore, it has been found that many MSM are also married and therefore put their spouses at high risk of being infected with HIV.

There is only limited information available in Nepal as regards prisoners and their vulnerability to HIV/STI. But worldwide (injecting) drug use, and sex (either between men or sexual harassment in female prisons) are common. As there is no access to condoms and/or sterile injection equipment, HIV, once introduced into the prison community, may spread quite rapidly. Moreover, most prisons are overcrowded and poor hygiene is a risk factor for all communicable diseases.

Young people (10-24 years) constitute 32 per cent of the total population of Nepal but Nepal's national HIV/AIDS/STI response has not sufficiently prioritised them as a primary target audience. Recent behavioural data indicate the increasing vulnerability of young people to HIV/AIDS in terms of a widening generational and cultural gap between emerging new values, (group) norms, knowledge and independence on the side of adolescents, and the values, reference points and norms on the side of the older generation. Girls, with their traditionally lower social status sometimes have knowledge about STDs and HIV/AIDS, but no access to any means of protection.

A KAPS survey among 1400 young people in seven different districts of Nepal 7 shows that Nepalese teenagers are highly aware of the HIV risk but that this awareness does not necessarily translate into safe sexual behaviour. Although an overwhelming majority of teenagers have heard of HIV/AIDS, only 74 per cent of teenagers knew that they should use condoms when having sex and only two-thirds said that they should not have sex with commercial sex workers.

The study also shows that almost 20 per cent of teenagers considered premarital sex as proper. One in five boys and nearly one in 10 girls interviewed had a sexual experience. 65 per cent of boys said that they had used condoms; while 74 per cent of girls said that their partners used a condom during sexual intercourse. Unprotected sex led to a 14 per cent pregnancy rate and a 22 per cent sexually transmitted diseases (STD) infection rate in boys and 13 per cent rate in girls. Pregnancy rates were high in districts where girls were pressured into having sex. The number of boys who had sex was far higher than the number of girls. Furthermore, the survey showed that 13 per cent had taken drugs, although only 5.4 per cent injected the drugs.

The national strategy therefore contains elements that move beyond providing youth with basic knowledge. It also strives to strengthen the skills of young people in decision-making, communication with their partners, negotiation of safe health behaviour, and anticipation of high-risk situations. It further recognises the need to help young people to develop their self-esteem and their ability to contribute through their active involvement in programming activities. Interventions can only be effective if they move beyond individual knowledge and encourage group norms for safe healthy behaviour. While it is important to continue activities that offer a basic knowledge about HIV/AIDS, as young people approach the age where they might become sexually active, it is equally important that messages be refined to address common misconceptions and gaps in knowledge identified by research.

In order to achieve empowerment of young people to voice their concerns and needs and to be included in decision making, key areas of intervention have been identified: ensuring an appropriate policy framework; the use of traditional and non-traditional mass media; and youth friendly services.

Following are preventing factors to HIV infection among young people:

i) Creating a supportive policy and community environment.
ii) Awareness and behaviour change communication.
iii) Youth-friendly services.
iv) Enhance young people's knowledge about HIV/AIDS/STI in formal and non-formal education settings.

In order to translate knowledge into practice, a supportive environment is needed for young people to protect themselves from HIV/AIDS/STI. The first priority therefore is to give young people a "voice" and to establish mechanisms through which this voice can be heard. Policy makers and communities should have accurate and relevant information about young people's issues and needs and include them in decision making around developing a youth-friendly environment and policy.

SOCIAL AWARENESS

Creating awareness among young people about HIV/AIDS/STI and reproductive health is a crucial first step for behaviour change. But awareness alone is not sufficient for behaviour change to occur. Therefore interventions need to be designed and targeted at empowering young people to have the knowledge, skills and the will to change their behaviour, and providing access to means of protection.

Strategies

i) Increase the use of mass and non-traditional media to promote safe sexual norms and healthy behaviour among young people including the options of consistent condom use, abstinence and delayed sexual activity.

ii) Empowerment of young people, particularly girls, in decisions regarding their sexual and reproductive lives through a life skills approach.

iii) Develop and implement programmes with full participation of young people to support young people's development and a healthy lifestyle.

iv) Expand quality peer education programmes for young people by building capacity of implementing organisations.

v) Increasing information and education activities (IEC) for recruits of uniformed services.

vi) Support and expand social marketing of behaviour change, including safer sex practices, through NGOs and private sector by:

vii) focusing on young people, especially those most at risk and uniformed services

viii) increasing the availability and accessibility of condoms · Promote condoms within family planning networks as the only method with a dual benefit of being able to prevent both HIV/ STDs and unwanted pregnancies.

Youth friendly services in Nepal are virtually non-existent. Information for young people comes mainly from peers and family members. In order to reduce the vulnerability of young people services including information must be tailored to their needs. The implementation of youth friendly services will have to start at selected locations with a view to future expansion.

HIV/AIDS: EDUCATION SETTINGS

Information provided through the formal and non-formal education settings plays an important role in supporting the other priorities defined in this chapter. Moreover, addressing HIV/AIDS/STI in educational settings can bring about positive changes in the immediate environment of young people.

Strategies

i) Development of an age-appropriate 'healthy life styles' curriculum, including basic information about HIV/AIDS and sex education.

ii) Include basic information on HIV/AIDS and reproductive health in the teacher's training and strengthen the capacity of teachers to deliver this information in an effective way.

iii) Involve NGOs in teacher training particularly in relation to young people's health, development and protection.

iv) Strengthen coordination and cooperation between key stakeholders in educational settings under the leadership of the Ministry of Education.

v) Incorporate HIV/AIDS/STI into the curriculum of Non-Formal Education and educational/training activities of employers and trade-unions.

CARE AND SUPPORT

Care and support for people living with HIV/AIDS has not been a prioritised part of the national response to the epidemic. However, given the increasing number of people infected and affected by HIV, this strategy will place more emphasis on care, support and basic treatment options. Stigma against and misconceptions about people living with HIV/AIDS currently inhibits access to what limited services are available. The specific needs of groups vulnerable to HIV/STI have not been addressed sufficiently by health and support services, in part because the users of these services have not been involved in their design.

Services and resources for confidential HIV testing, counselling, laboratory investigations, treatment, care and support have been inadequate in terms of coverage and quality. Training and guidelines for health workers regarding counselling, care and treatment of those infected and affected by HIV/AIDS have been lacking. Similarly little support is available to help those caring for people living with HIV/AIDS within families and communities.

The priorities include:

i) Reducing stigma surrounding people living with HIV/AIDS
ii) Voluntary confidential counselling and testing for selected groups
iii) Prevention of mother to child transmission for known cases
iv) Community and home based care and support
v) Standard treatment guidelines
vi) Media services.

Reducing stigma surrounding people living with HIV/AIDS is a crucial first step towards not only improving the uptake of support services such as voluntary counselling and HIV testing but also increasing acceptance within society.

Strategies

i) The use of mass media featuring political and religious leaders as well as celebrities to break down the barriers surrounding IV/AIDS like exclusion, misconceptions and denial.
ii) Ensure that Nepal's legal and policy environment does not represent a barrier to the acceptance and integration of people infected and affected by HIV/AIDS into society.

iii) Ensure that legal and policy environment allows people living with HIV/AIDS to attain their full human rights and that there is no barrier to increased acceptance of these people.

iv) Strengthen the ability of people living with AIDS to organise themselves and to effective voice issues that are of concern to them through:
   a) support groups
   b) leadership training
   c) legal support

v) Ensure the full involvement of people living with HIV/AIDS in the decision process at all levels of policy and programme development, implementation and monitoring.

vi) Ensure that policies are in place and implemented focusing on HIV/AIDS and the workpalce.

vii) Ensure all HIV/AIDS/STI prevention programmes include activities aimed at reducing stigma.

Confidential Counselling

Voluntary confidential counselling and HIV testing is a key entry point for care and support services as well as helping individual decision-making. Nepal will adopt a phased approach, as defined by the following key strategies, in order to reach the objective. In a first phase, VCT services will be implemented focusing on selected groups (sex workers, clients, injecting drug users, labour migrants, uniformed services and their respective partners). At a later stage it will be expanded to focus on young people and the general population.

Strategies

i) develop a policy and quality framework for government and private institutions, including NGOs, in relation to HIV testing and counselling procedures by:

ii) developing a national protocol on HIV testing and counselling including a reference system according to the current WHO-recommended criteria;

iii) developing counselling criteria including training, supervision and monitoring; and establishing quality assurance and control mechanisms for HIV testing and counselling.

iv) ensure that no HIV testing contravenes with either the constitution or the law.

v) design and gradually implement VCT services based on prioritised needs focusing on sex workers, clients, injecting drug users, labour migrants, uniformed services and their respective partners.

v) expand VCT services based on the prioritised needs of other groups starting with young people

vi) provide public information about the importance of voluntary counselling and testing and the right to confidentiality.

Community Home-based Care

Community home-based care acknowledges that care and support is much more than medical treatment. It is seen as the basis for any support system for people infected and affected by HIV/AIDS. The prerequisite for community and home-based care is that those infected and affected are fully accepted by and integrated into their respective environment.

Strategies

i) Develop information material about community and home-based care describing possible roles of the family, community and service providers to provide support to people infected and affected including palliative care.

ii) Support the establishment of support networks at different levels for people infected and affected by HIV/AIDS.

iii) Build capacity among government and non-government programmes who have an existing relationship with communities in order to inform and motivate communities for home-based care and support.

iv) Ensure the health care providers have the capacity to provide basic care and counselling services. Priority will be given to the most affected areas.

v) Develop a policy framework regarding mechanism for government institutions to involve NGOs or other organisations in proving services to people infected and affected by HIV/AIDS.

vi) Develop a policy framework for orphans and children in families made vulnerable by HIV/AIDS.

Medical Services

In a resource poor setting like Nepal, immediate universal access to anti-retroviral therapy and certain other AIDS-related medical interventions is not possible. However, every effort must be put into building up a system of effective medical care, providing a basis for future treatment options.

Strategies

i) Develop a standard treatment protocol that:

ii) includes treatment, mental health care, terminal care ensures that treatment is initiated based on the recommendation of trained health personnel;

iii) describes a referral system

iv) Ensure that drugs to treat opportunistic infections are included in the essential drug list and are available.

v) Design and implement a quality control/assurance system to monitor medical services both in public and private sectors as regards to HIV/AIDS.

vi) Establish regional centres at locations that provide equitable access for all people in Nepal. Each of those centres should be able to provide diagnosis, treatment and care for HIV/AIDS, related illnesses and STDs. It should therefore have adequate staffing, laboratory and X-ray facilities.

vii) Ensure confidential services at all levels, through training of staff and regular follow-up.

viii) Establish a reporting and information system preferably using existing structures.

Nepal's surveillance system for HIV has improved but remains inadequate in tracking the epidemic in all risk groups. An emphasis on male patients symptomatic for sexually transmitted infections as a marker for risk groups meant that the sentinel surveillance missed the recent dramatic increase in HIV prevalence amongst sex workers and injecting drug users. Moreover the results of many HIV tests conducted in hospitals and private clinics are not reported to the NCASC and research on HIV has not been well coordinated and/or prioritised and ethical questions have been raised about some of the research protocols.

IMPLEMENTATION OF EXPANDED RESPONSE TO HIV/AIDS

The main challenge for Nepal is to respond immediately to a rapidly evolving HIV/AIDS epidemic. This has to be undertaken in the context of a civil conflict in the country 8, weak implementation capacity both within the public and the private sector, structural weaknesses with respect to multi-sector involvement, coordination, policy, monitoring and evaluation, and scarce internal resources.

Recognising all the above, Nepal has embarked to broaden and to deepen political commitment. For example, establishing the National AIDS Council under the chairmanship of the Rt. Honourable Prime Minister, defining HIV/AIDS as priority "1" in the MTEP of the MoH and integrating HIV/AIDS in the 10th Development Plan. HMG is also committed to reforming and strengthening the management mechanisms of an expanded, i.e. multi-sector and scaled-up, response to HIV/AIDS within the framework of the National Strategy.

The challenge will be to sustain and to broaden the political commitment in terms of policy, involvement of new partners and stakeholders, and finally also to translate political commitment and leadership into action. As a resource poor country with additional security expenses, it is difficult for Nepal to demonstrate commitment through budgetary allocations, but higher allocations to an expanded response are foreseen in the MTEP of the MoH. The recent active involvement of lawmakers and municipalities both in the strategy development and in policy issues signals broadening commitment that goes beyond parties.

The strategy tries throughout to address the issue of commitment, enabling environment at all levels, and local ownership. It seeks to increase the understanding of decision-makers and communities, especially as regards the most vulnerable groups, and to actively involve them in the response. In doing so, a broader base of commitment will be established and ultimately facilitate the implementation of the strategy. The involvement of local communities and authorities will also contribute to a public accountability as regards the implementation of the strategy.

Ideally, the National Strategy will be "programme" funded, i.e. pooled resources and/or earmarked contributions, to provide required resources. The future management and implementation structures will be designed to:

i) Support and strengthen the leading role of government, and the MoH as the technical line ministry, as regards: policy and strategy; monitoring and evaluation, including quality assurance and quality control; epidemiology and surveillance; involvement of other government structures, e.g. other line ministries, and coordination;

ii) Provide the flexibility, accountability and results oriented management of a larger programme at the central and the decentralised level;
iii) Establish new public-private partnerships at all levels to fight the epidemic;
iv) De-medicalise the response to HIV/AIDS;
v) Support decentralisation and integration at the community level;
vi) Increase responsiveness; and,
vii) Provide the basis for sustainability through the involvement of the private sector and civil society.

The shift from individually funded "projects" to a "programme", from outputs to results orientation, from donor interest to national priorities, from capacity building of central structures to strengthening of implementation capacity, and from a health sector response to a multi-sector approach will require time and resources. This is, however, the precondition for an effective and efficient national response. Finally, in order to respond effectively, financial and human resources will be needed to translate the national strategy into action. As the epidemic advances day by day, the overall resource requirements to respond become bigger and bigger. Nepal will need the support by external development partners to fulfil the resource needs.

The strategy addresses sustainability in providing for innovative financing mechanisms, and in strengthening the capacity and empowering vulnerable groups and communities. It is hoped that involvement of communities, decentralisation, and integration in development programmes will also contribute to better sustainability.

The following is an outline of a "vision", which in the process of operationalising and reviewing may change. Based on "lessons learned" in Nepal and other countries, it reflects the will and commitment of Nepal to respond to the epidemic.

A dynamic public-private partnership charged with managing and implementing an expanded response to HIV/AIDS in Nepal.

Weak management at all levels may seriously affect the implementation of the national strategy. The experience of the past was frequently changing key-staff in line ministries, slow government procedures, and sometimes lack of transparency and accountability.

The change to result oriented management (and this means primarily implementation), out sourcing of defined parts of the strategy to a private entity with appropriate capacity, ensuring transparency and accountability through a trust fund mechanism, and restructuring of the NCASC to the technical wing of an expanded response will secure the competence and flexibility needed to respond quickly and effectively.

The modification of the NACC to an executive public-private body overseeing the implementation of the national strategy will in itself ensure broader involvement of key-stake holders and will put the focus on implementation.

National AIDS Council

With the establishment of the National AIDS Council under the chair of the Prime Minister, Nepal has set the stage for the highest possible leadership. The multi-sector composition of the council will allow for greater involvement of different ministries, the private sector and civil society, and will serve as an important advocacy body.

The National AIDS Council will review and approve national policies and strategies and will be involved in advocacy and monitoring the implementation of the strategy.

Establishment of a public-private partnership at central level for policy, programme decisions, monitoring and evaluation, coordination, and financial allocation for the operationalisation of the National Strategy.

The National AIDS Coordination Committee (NACC) originally included representatives of all line ministries, NGOs, the private sector and donors. In order to improve its efficiency and to make it the executive body to oversee the implementation of the National Strategy, the composition was reviewed and the new NACC will have 12 members: 4 government representatives, 2 representatives from the private sector, 4 NGO representatives (including PLWHA), 1 bilateral donor and 1 multilateral organisation.

The NACC will act as a "board of directors" to the Nepal Trust Fund, and will be responsible for reviewing and approving workplans and budgets, reviewing reports, and guiding implementation of the national strategy. The NCASC will have the technical review authority and will advise the board of directors on policy and funding issues. The NACC will report to the NAC.

The Minister of Health will chair the NACC. The NCASC will act as the secretariat to the NACC. The NACC will be the governing body of the Nepal Trust Fund and will:

i) Set policies and strategies for the Fund consistent with the agreed Purpose, Principles and Scope;

ii) Set operational guidelines, and budgets for the NCASC and the private entity executing the programme;

iii) Approve workplans and budgets;

iv) Appoint and, if necessary, replace the Executive Head of the private entity;

v) Set criteria for membership of advisory groups as appropriate;

vi) Establish a framework for monitoring and periodic independent evaluation of performance and financial accountability of activities supported by the Fund;

vii) Consider, approve, and monitor cooperative arrangements or agreements with other organisations and institutions;

viii) Represent the views of the various constituencies;

ix) Act as the main coordination mechanism for an expanded response;

x) Advocate for the Fund, and mobilise resources.

A future programme approach requires the establishment of adequate fund flow mechanisms both to government and to private (non-government) institutions. This will be done through the establishment of a Trust Fund. The purpose of the Fund is to attract, manage and disburse resources for an expanded response to HIV/AIDS in Nepal through a new public-private partnership. This partnership will strengthen services and participation of all strata of society and make a sustainable and significant contribution to the reduction of infections, illness and death, and thereby mitigate the impact caused by HIV/AIDS and STIs. The trust fund will provide resources for the implementation of the National Strategy for government and non-government partners. It will be governed by the NACC.

Restructuring and strengthening of the NCASC as the "technical authority" in Nepal as regards to evidence based policy/strategy, research, monitoring and evaluation, epidemiology and surveillance, STD, and technical assistance to government, e.g. line ministries, DDCs.

The National Centre for AIDS and STD Control (NCASC) will be restructured and strengthened to act as the technical authority for the national programme with the following key functions:

The NCASC reports to the NACC, and will advise the NACC on technical aspects of policy, strategy, and programme execution/implementation. The NCASC will prepare annual workplans and budgets to be approved by the NACC. Resources for the core functions of the NCASC will come from the national budget and, if needed, from the trust fund. Establishment of a private entity to execute the programme within the framework of the National Strategy, and the objectives of the 10th Five Year Plan and MTEP respectively.

Acknowledging that the private sector (including NGOs) and civil society play a crucial role in an expanded response, the execution of the National Strategy, especially in areas where government has either no specific interfaces or capacity will be out-sourced to a newly established private entity and monitored by the NCASC and the NACC respectively. This private entity will, under the leadership of the NCASC, develop annual workplans and budgets. It will be guided by the board, and by yearly targets set by the NCASC and other national authorities.

Based on these results oriented workplans, which will address priorities defined in the National Strategy, the private entity will call for proposals from implementing partners. Proposals and capacity of implementing partners will be reviewed and will be integrated in the workplan, thus forming an annual programme. The programme will also identify necessary areas for capacity building among implementing partners, and will facilitate and support new partnerships at all levels.

Technical assistance to implementing partners will be provided, if needed, both for the development of proposals, and for actual implementation. In this regard, the private entity will only facilitate, broker and resource the needed technical assistance. The board and the NCASC will review the programme, and funds will be released to the entity after approval by the board. The board of directors will set the operational guidelines, approve workplans and budget and will appoint the CEO. The entity will be staffed with 5-7 professionals and adequate support staff.

The main functions of this private entity are to:

i) Prepare annual workplans, budgets and quarterly reports to be approved by the board (NACC);
ii) Manage all aspects of subcontracts to implementing partners;
iii) Establish a technical review panel and ensure the independence of the review process;

iv) Coordinate with all relevant agencies, especially with the director NCASC;

v) Facilitate and support technical assistance to implementing partners;

vi) Communicate the board's decisions to stakeholders;

vii) Support the board in advocacy and fund raising.

Development of district strategies to respond to HIV/AIDS at the decentralised level and the establishment of appropriate management bodies at the District level. The National Strategy provides the overall guiding framework for an expanded response at the decentralised level. In order to support districts and communities to identify issues of their concern and to develop adequate responses within the framework of the national strategy, the facilitation and support to the development of District strategies is seen as a priority area of the National Strategy.

Ultimately the national strategy has to be translated into a programme with concrete actions. The biggest risk for not achieving the goals of the strategy (and thus failing to stop the epidemic) lies in the weak implementation and management capacity at all levels. Although the strengthening of implementation and management capacities are priority areas of the national strategy, the challenge is to balance implementation and "central" capacity needs in order to start activities in a quality and quantity necessary to produce impact on the epidemic.

This will be achieved through a programme approach, which will focus on the priority areas of the national strategy and combines implementation with strengthening of needed capacities. The expanded response is therefore not a combination of individual projects, but a carefully designed and managed partnership approach. Using synergies and comparative advantages of different actors, actively promoting partnerships, providing technical assistance to implementing partners, and improved coordination are defined key-strategies and will enable a rapid scaling up of activities.

REFERENCES

Government of Nepal, Strategic Plan for HIV and AIDS in Nepal 1997-2001, Final Draft, July, 2002.

Human Development Repot, 2001.

NCASC, Situational Analysis of HIV/AIDS in Nepal, NCASC, Ministry of Health, Kathmandu, December, 2000.

8

Assessment of Maldives

The Maldives, a small unique South Asian island nation of about 277,000 people, has to date enjoyed relative freedom from the HIV pandemic. Although some 84 documented cases (as of June 2000) are known, the majority of these have been expatriates or Maldivians with a history of travel abroad, such as sailors. This is an expected pattern. In almost all nations, the virus has been brought in through such mechanisms. Eventually, however, internal transmission usually ensues. The threat of continued growth in HIV prevalence in the Maldives depends on the proportion of people engaging in unprotected sex with infected partners, its spread to pregnant women and their babies, and the proportion exposed to unsafe blood-related procedures. While strict religious principles may appear to be protective, HIV is simply a virus and does not distinguish whether the sex act through which it is spread is a moral or immoral, legal or illegal act. Hence, the risks of an epidemic cannot be viewed in terms of the frequency of socially approved vs. socially disapproved sexual behaviour; rather it must be assessed in epidemiological terms as these relate to the frequency of sexual partner change and the sexual networks thereby created.

Transmission from mother to child usually follows as the second most common route of transmission when the prevalence of HIV reaches about 3-5 per cent in high risk groups and begins moving into the general population. Transmission via blood accounts for a smaller proportion of all cases, less than 10 per cent worldwide. Blood-related transmission is seldom a major mode of spread, except in the case of injecting drug users (IDUs). HIV is still an emerging epidemic and spreading more widely and rapidly than previously expected. In Middle Eastern nations, where overall prevalence has been low, there are now high levels among IDUs. The same pattern is unfolding in Pakistan and Indonesia. In nation after nation, the proportion of females becoming infected is rising, in many cases because they are the partners of IDUs or men who have sex with men (MSM) or purchase sex from female sex workers.

The major risk factor for women who acquire HIV in India now is simply being married. HIV finds the cracks in society and follows them. Poor health services, inequitable gender relations, governmental corruption, poverty, war, unstable family life, high fertility, unemployment, high levels of mobility, ignorance—these and many more factors play a role in the HIV pandemic. Any analysis of the HIV situation in a country is in fact an analysis of the social and institutional development of that country. Preventing an HIV epidemic requires far more than dealing with the virus as a pathogen. It requires knowing and understanding the social and environmental conditions that contribute to people's vulnerability to exposure. These include all the factors that make it difficult for people to protect themselves even when they know full well what the virus is, how it is transmitted and that it is invariably fatal. It has been shown repeatedly that knowledge of HIV is not sufficient to provide protection. Prevention programmes must be properly tailored to meet the social realities of a given society. Where denial and stigma reign, these must be defeated.

In recognition of the need to assess the social and behavioural risk factors for HIV, as well as the responses to date, the Government of Maldives, in cooperation with the UN Theme Group and with financial support from UNICEF and the Resident Coordinator Funds, requested an independent assessment, to be followed by recommendations to address the issues raised. On 6 th June, 2000, the consultant undertook this assignment, which was completed on the 29 th June. Assessing risk factors under such short-term assignment conditions can, at best, yield an imprecise, qualitative overview.

More accurate predictions or modelling of the potential epidemic in the Maldives cannot be undertaken without quantitative data on the prevalence of sexually transmitted diseases and the prevalence and intensity of behavioural risk factors, particularly among high risk groups. Assessing gaps in prevention services is somewhat more achievable. However, well-planned and designed HIV prevention programmes require the specific targeting of known high risk groups, particularly during the early stages of the epidemic. Hence, even gaps in prevention cannot properly be assessed without evidence as to which groups might be considered most vulnerable, the sizes of these groups and how they may be reached. Because such data are not available at present, this assessment has attempted to construct a likely scenario based on the following sources of information, collected within Male' and during visits to atolls in the north, central and southern regions:

i) A review of documents relating to social and economic issues bearing on health in general, and specifically on reproductive health and HIV;

ii) Interviews with persons representing agencies within and outside of government having particular knowledge of HIV/AIDS and/or reproductive health;

iii) Interviews with persons from sub-sectors of society thought to be at relatively increased risk of acquiring an HIV infection. The information gathered from these sources is synthesised around focal issues of importance to assess the level of risk among individuals and the potential to sustain an epidemic. Where relevant, any responses carried out in the country are then recounted and the justification for doing more or less in the short, medium or long term is discussed.

Due to the sensitive nature of some of the information sought, most interviews were conducted in private and without interpreters, necessitating at least simple English-speaking ability on the part of respondents. Where this was not possible, small focus group discussions were held using interpreters. As the focus group discussion is not a suitable technique for acquiring information on sensitive or hidden issues, it should be recognised that some information is likely to have been under-reported and false. This problem was handled through triangulation with as many sources of information as could be found in a short period of time

ISSUES OF VULNERABILITY

The nation of Maldives, despite severe challenges, has demonstrated remarkable success in a number of important social, economic and health indicators over the past three decades. In terms of indicators immediately pertinent to the usual risks for HIV, literacy, educational coverage, the provision of health care facilities, GDP, acceptance of family planning, life expectancy, and maternal mortality have all shown marked improvements. Progressive action with regard to a number of other health and social issues has been instituted, such as hepatitis B immunisation, drug abuse de-addiction services and others. There are, however, areas for concern with regard to income disparity, gender inequality, information restriction, crowding, unemployment, and others. These factors are all variously linked to high levels of mobility, both within the country and outside of it. Migrants are always at greater risk due to loneliness, fewer mechanisms of social control when away from home and general anomie. These factors are also associated with increasing drug abuse among the youth, which in turn may be associated with increased sexual risk taking.

The demographic profile of a rapidly increasing young population in an environment with foreseeable economic limitations sets the stage for a potentially disruptive set of social changes frequently associated with the spread of HIV. The numbers of cases of HIV detected to date cannot depict the epidemic's potential. Wisdom dictates preparedness based on a careful analysis of available information and the generation of accurate, appropriate behavioural information that will provide the basis for a national programme of HIV/AIDS/STD prevention.

ECONOMIC FACTORS

Personal incomes have risen considerably in the Maldives over the past few decades as tourism and fishing have become lucrative sources of national wealth. Increased government spending on education and health have yielded considerable improvement in basic amenities, such as potable water, sanitation, primary health services, and literacy, but a recent study shows that about 15 per cent of the population lives on less than Rf 7.5 (US$0.65) per person per day, with the highest concentration of low incomes in Male'. As the centre of gravity for development for all of the Maldives, Male' exhibits the greatest income disparity. With about 27 per cent of the nation's population living on 1.8 sq km of land, crowding and its attendant high prices are extreme on Male'. Such relative differences in wealth have well-known detrimental social effects, particularly on youth.

Exposure to the consumerism of mass media and over-reliance on formal education can combine to raise expectations of material wellbeing to unrealistic levels, leading to resentful and socially deviant behaviour. Income disparity and a sense of relative deprivation produce gradual changes in the social fabric that reduce the impact of normative mechanisms of social control, such as religious principles, family cohesiveness, and the authority of community leaders. Unplanned urbanisation and crowding on Male' contributes significantly to general interpersonal stress.

Although the rate of population increase has dropped from 3.4 per cent in 1990 to 2.8 per cent in 1995, a projected population size of .5 million by the year 2020 will seriously stress the nation's resources. All of these factors emanate from an economic situation of considerable vulnerability and insecurity. This creates the backdrop for a predictable increase in risk-taking behaviour, particularly among youth.

Mobility

Mobility, both in and out of the Maldives, is a feature of life affecting many families. There are about 24,000 foreign workers in the country, 90 per cent of whom are male. About 10,000 live and work on Male' alone. The sex ratio on Male' as of 1995 was 2.2:1 males to females. Others are mostly employed at resorts and in construction and garment factories scattered about the islands. For a variety of reasons, Maldivians cannot fill all the employment needs of the country, despite being in need of employment themselves. Lower level domestic service jobs, mostly in Male; are being filled by Indian and Sri Lankan maid servants and many jobs in shops, restaurants and construction by Bangladeshi, Indian and Sri Lankan men. Garment factories employ a small number of local women, but also bring in women from China and elsewhere with known skills in the industry.

Expatriate workers also often fill positions in teaching and medicine. In most nations, this type of migrant labour has led to the growth of prostitution to serve these men. Migrant female domestic workers may also be vulnerable either to coerced or commercial sex. There is considerable anecdotal evidence that such a trade exists in the Maldives, especially in Male' where a floating population of thousands contributes to the anonymity necessary for an illicit trade.

Due to the lack of educational facilities, numerous Maldivian students go abroad for higher education. For shorter periods, many Maldivians go abroad for business or to seek health care or other services not available in the Maldives. Many thousands go to Male' from the atolls to attend school or for shorter-term purposes. This constant movement of people implies some level of risk for HIV and may require specialised prevention programmes. About 2000 men serve as seamen, mainly on international cargo vessels. The number has been halved in the past few years. These seamen represent a high risk group by virtue of their occupational conditions and subculture.

Tourism

Tourism accounts for the main source of national income, but is thought to bring certain problems as well. The main issues that relate to HIV risk appear to be the exposure of Maldivians to lifestyles other than their own and the long separation of men from their families. The movement of men to work on islands other than their homes is a relatively new demographic phenomenon within the Maldives. There are at least 84 designated tourist islands that remain separate from inhabited islands according to government policy. Few women are involved in the tourist industry as workers, less than 100 out of about 5000 in 1996.

All-male residential groups are crowded and many have insufficient shower/toilet facilities for these men. Some inhabited islands have a large number of men away most of the time working at resorts, such as Addu Atoll which had a residential ratio of men per woman in 1995 of 0.83. Men working at resorts may, if the distance is not great, return frequently, but more commonly, visits to families take place only quarterly within the year or even less often. Foreign men on contract can return to their homes only once every two years. Such migratory conditions create considerable vulnerability for the sexual transmission of HIV. Long separated periods, of course, strain marriage relationships and many women consider that the lack of male discipline in the home has led to greater misbehaviour of their children. The stress and isolation of living in crowded all-male groups at resort islands contributes to HIV risk.

Sexual relations between males and between male workers and female tourists are known to take place at the resorts.

Recourse to commercial sex in Male; 'has been reported for some unknown proportion of these men and expert informants consider that the greatest risk for Maldivian men emanates from conditions on Male', not from the resort tourist. As the Maldives is not a destination for sex tourists, the great majority of clientele at the resorts are not likely to be persons having sexually transmitted infections, such as HIV.

The nations from which the majority of tourists come, i.e. Italy, Germany, Switzerland, Japan, are not generally high HIV prevalence nations. As of 1997, the prevalence of AIDS cases per 100,000 was highest in Switzerland (83.8), followed by Italy (71.5), and Germany (20.7). Japan has very low AIDS prevalence (1.2). These figures do not reflect current HIV prevalence, but as of the end of 1999, this was 0.25 for Western Europe as a whole, less than half of that for South East and South Asia or North America. Rates of HIV incidence (numbers of new infections) are far higher for South Asia than for Western Europe. A large proportion of the epidemic in European countries has been due to the early spread among gay men and injecting drug users. While the transfer of HIV from a tourist to a Maldivian resort worker certainly might occur, the likelihood of HIV reaching epidemic proportions via this source seems extremely low. Of greater importance is the indigenous transmission of HIV among Maldivians, should HIV have a chance to accumulate in any one at-risk group.

SOCIAL FACTORS

Gender discrimination is less pronounced in the Maldives than in many other nations in the South Asian region, a region in which such discrimination is extreme by world standards. Government's efforts to equalise opportunities for male and female children have been considerable and show impact. Differential advantages, however, are evident in several important areas, largely driven by traditional cultural practices and attitudes. Girl children are raised to be more shy and compliant and carry a larger role in daily household responsibilities than boys. On the islands, their mobility is constrained to the extent that, after attaining adulthood, such simple activities as swimming are seen to be unseemly.

Although one in three households is headed by women, largely by their own declaration, women are under-represented in the labour force and a higher proportion of women wish to work than can find work. Generally, they are prevented from working by parents and husbands (1,10). Women's proportional role in productive economic activities has diminished with increasing tourism and changes in the fishing industry over the past several decades that have reduced the profitability of drying fish, dropping from 60 per cent in 1977 to 20 per cent in 1990 (1). Recently, this rate appears to have risen to about 25 per cent. However, on Male', women's employment has greatly increased relative to that on the atolls over the years. Nonetheless, 70 per cent of government jobs were still held by men as of 1998.

The lack of labour participation among women is largely due to constrained mobility relative to men and to lesser achievement in higher secondary education. Generally, however, girls perform at least as well in school as do boys and, with the exception of grades 10-12, are approximately equally represented. Violence against women as well as sexual abuse of girls and women are under-reported and as such, are left largely unattended as social problems. Recent attention to child abuse has resulted in rising numbers of reported cases, including that of sexual abuse. Women's rights are less well protected than men's in divorce and less than half of women with children receive financial support from their ex-husbands, as required by law. Legal rights and political positions for women are areas yet to be expanded.

The social fact that one must obey one's husband or risk divorce is frequently stated by women, but does not seem to be as great a constraint on behaviour as it is elsewhere in South Asia. Some women claim that their husbands only, not they, can access condoms from family health workers, though health workers dispute this. Overall, compared to their sisters of similar economic status in India and Bangladesh, Maldivian women are better-off in terms of social, health and educational indicators. But, whatever social or cultural factors exist that create power differentials between the genders such that a woman would have greater difficulty protecting herself from exposure to HIV, these contribute to the steadily rising proportion of infection among females in the world today. If these are operative in Maldivian personal life, they will produce the same effect.

Monogamy, as distinguished from serial monogamy, is the marital union of a couple for life. In monogamous societies, the most frequent cause of marital dissolution is the death of a spouse. Serial monogamy, on the other hand, is distinguished by high levels of divorce and remarriage. Historical records demonstrate that serial monogamy is an old cultural pattern, well documented for at least 400 years and found in the neighbouring atolls of Laccadives and Kerala as well. The age at first marriage for women as of 1990 was 16.5, but there are recent indications of an increase to about 17.9 in younger women. Men are married at around the age of 20-21. In 1970 divorce statistics showed 85 divorces for every 100 marriages; this dropped to 70 per 100 in 1990. Only 8 per cent of marriages ended through the death of a spouse. Studies have been conducted or information compiled to seek an understanding of this pattern.

Although efforts to diminish the ease at which men can acquire divorce focus on Islamic legal rights, the cultural pattern of early marriage with rapid remarriage predates the conversion to Islam in the Maldives. A proportion of remarriages takes place among the same couples who were once divorced, so that women end up having 3 to 4 marriages to 2 to 3 men. On Male', women as well as men seek divorce fairly frequently, unlike on the atolls. Divorced women are not stigmatised. Similar marriage patterns averaging 40-50 per cent divorce rates are found in non-Islamic atoll societies in the Pacific as well and may be more related to the constrictions of atoll life and matrilineal social structures than to Islam. Until recently, Maldivians do not seem to have considered this a serious social problem. In terms of modern concepts of reproductive and family health, the problems in such marriage patterns relate to:

i) possible detrimental effects on children,
ii) possibly acting as a driving force for high fertility and
iii) the frequency of sexual partner change.

With respect to HIV, the issue to be considered is whether such a marriage pattern allows a high level of overall partner change, with overlapping concurrent partners. As HIV has a long silent period, one infected man (or woman) could conceivably infect several spouses before showing signs of AIDS. Particularly for the first few marriages, time periods between partners may be quite short, with one document reporting 20 per cent of marriages becoming divorced in less than one year. In another study, 21 per cent of both men and women queried gave infidelity as the reason for divorce. If these statistics correctly describe high levels of concurrent partners, then high levels of divorce could be seen as an indicator of risk behaviours supportive of an HIV epidemic. There are other factors to consider.

i) Recently, with increased education and modernisation, divorce rates appear to be diminishing, in direct contrast to patterns in developed nations, such as the USA (17).
ii) Marriage patterns remain largely endogamous (among persons from the same island) for the first marriage (57 per cent) but become increasingly less so with subsequent marriages.

As elsewhere, women generally marry men older than themselves and the age gap also increases with subsequent marriages. Thus, the sexual networks in which married people are involved are under change, with both positive and negative forces present with regard to their ability to drive an HIV epidemic. Overall rates of sexual partner change remain the more important and easily documented determinant of HIV epidemics. These are far greater wherever sex is commercialised or commodified. If HIV were to rise to 2-5 per cent in a group of women selling sex to divorced or separated men, then the pattern of serial monogamy could become a cultural feature contributing to the spread of HIV. At the present time, without knowing the rates of casual sex that accompanies such a marriage pattern, it is impossible to estimate the risks involved. However, spread through such a mechanism is far more likely than is the accumulation of cases needed to sustain an epidemic.

SEXUAL BEHAVIOUR

All sexual behaviours that spread HIV are found in the Maldives, but the frequencies and numbers of persons involved are yet unknown. Foreign and Maldivian sex workers can be found in Male', as can standard South Asian patterns of homosexuality. Large numbers of male workers away from their homes create a pool of potential commercial sex clients. Maldivian men as well as expatriate men frequent sex workers but what proportion of the general male population does so and how frequently are unknown. Key informants indicate that sexual networks among men who have sex with men (MSM) may be far larger than among men and women practising casual sex. Fears of discovery and legal prosecution may limit these practices, but do not diminish them entirely. Because ease of access to women appears to be more common in the Maldives than elsewhere in South Asia, dependence on sex workers, particularly among the young and unmarried, may be less frequent than in some neighbouring countries. This could prove to be a protective factor for HIV, in that fewer men may be likely to be exposed to women in whom HIV could easily reach high levels of prevalence, such as sex workers. But again, if HIV were to become concentrated to any extent among those who do sell sex, the spread from their clients to other women would be assured.

Youth always comprises a particularly vulnerable group for HIV. Maldives has a young population with about 47 per cent under 15 years old. These are the youngsters who will have to cope with the coming years of the epidemic and experts estimate that we are only about one-tenth through this pandemic of HIV. Those who are young and reaching ages now at which sexual activity is more likely, 15-25, comprise another 20 per cent of the population.

With a median age at first marriage of 17 among girls, at least 50 per cent will definitely be sexually active. Among those who are not married estimates of premarital sex guessed at by those interviewed for this exercise ranged from 50 per cent to 75 per cent. Whatever the reality may be, some proportion of young people experiment with sex before marriage and all will do so at some time. By the age of 21, the average age at marriage for young men, it is likely that a very high proportion will have had sexual intercourse at least once. AIDS prevention messages must accommodate the reality of young peoples' lives.

Parents and relatives do not teach anything about sex, sexual relationships, marriage, reproduction, STDs or related issues to their children. Neither the primary nor the secondary school curriculum covers more than the biological aspects of reproduction. Most young people report they learn about sex from other youth, sometimes siblings, and TV. Others say they learn from no one.

Despite the reality that satellite television brings the usual messages of commodified or casual sex and pornography is readily accessed on the Internet and elsewhere, no effort is made to provide alternate or complementary models of healthy, responsible sexuality. On many islands there are no book stores and it is doubtful if useful books on these topics can be easily found, even in Male'.

Family life skills or life skills education is not carried out by any NGOs, schools or government departments. Similarly, personnel working on AIDS prevention appear to have little or no access to up-to-date information on the epidemic, its epidemiology, the social and behavioural aspects of human sexuality, theory and practice in behavioural change, best practices in prevention programme design and execution, recommended surveillance methods, etc.

AIDS-related scientific journals are not apparently acquired by the Department of Public Health or any other agency. Suitable persons are often not selected to attend international meetings sponsored by WHO, UNAIDS, or others. Web-based information sources are still quite expensive to access and not frequently used in the Department of Public Health or in some of the UN agencies.

On Male', 48 per cent and in the atolls, 55 per cent of the population have no radio at home. The comparable figures for TV are 45 per cent and 86 per cent. Newspapers are transported to the islands but on an irregular basis. On Male' both newspapers and magazines are more widely available. Despite high levels of literacy, functional literacy is far lower. All media are subject to the national censorship board, except satellite TV and the Internet.

The nature of surveillance as case detection, as opposed to research to detect trends in infections and behaviours, does not lend itself to publication and dissemination. Public and official dissemination of the results of all the testing is extremely limited. This approach is counter to improving awareness and leads to mistaken rumours, sometimes in the direction of exaggerated numbers. Surprisingly, in an exercise conducted as part of the Master Health Plan, to rank health priorities through discussions with many stakeholders, AIDS ranked first.

The lack of accurate information amongst the public can also lead to a situation in which HIV is not taken as a serious threat and to a belief that caution is not necessary. The public's health is not well served by limiting the information available about HIV in their country or region. A recent survey on reproductive health reveals inadequate knowledge about STDs among health workers. About 31 per cent could name a symptom of STDs, but none mentioned that most STIs are asymptomatic, associated these with infertility, ectopic pregnancies or pelvic inflammatory disease (PID).

More than half (68 per cent) felt STDs were rare in their communities. It appears they assume the population rarely has STIs because few people come for treatment. Knowledge of the symptoms and consequences of STIs is similarly low among the general public, although many readily admit that such diseases exist in their community and that people go abroad for treatment. Due to widespread awareness campaigns and TV exposure, most of the public does know that HIV is a virus that is sexually transmitted and fatal. Fewer know it can be transmitted through blood contact and very few understand mother-to-child transmission.

A common misconception is that classic STDs, if left unattended, can develop into HIV. Few doctors know how HIV disease may present clinically in men and women nor are there treatment guidelines available for HIV disease, AIDS or the reduction of perinatal transmission. Some health workers and many lay people alike appear very interested in learning more about the biological aspects of STDs, including HIV.

As most people have no experience discussing sex and it does not appear that health workers are given training in taking a sexual history even in their pre-professional training, the social and behavioural aspects of STD counselling are nearly totally lacking. Except for two persons sent out for training (who are not now active in the programme), professional training in STD or HIV counselling has not taken place for health workers or others.

Drug Abuse

The epidemic of drug abuse is itself, in addition to HIV/AIDS, a major social and health problem in the entire South and South East Asian region. In the Maldives, given the lack of accurate information available, evidence gathered during this assessment points to drug abuse associated sexual behaviour among youth as the single most obvious potential risk factor for HIV. This is simply because the sale of sex for drug money (or the exchange of sex for drugs) is a more likely scenario than others to bring about frequent partner change and the potential for accumulation of HIV infections. The street price of a single piece (one dose) of heroin in Male' is relatively high at 100 Rf., 5 times the price in Bangladesh and India. Depending on the disposable income of young people, several doses per day could easily become a difficult financial strain.

Female sex workers, i.e. who make a living from selling sex on a regular basis, in most countries have between 200 (Indonesia) and 1000 (Cambodia) clients per year (though these may not all be different men). The chance of being exposed to HIV is so much greater among these women than women in all other situations. They, of course, acquire HIV from infected clients and can then infect other clients, if condoms are not consistently used. In most of South and South East Asia, professional sex workers are not generally regular drug abusers, as they are in, for example, New York. It is not known to what extent young female drug users in the Maldives are engaging in frequent partner change. It is clear, however, that the number of drug related offences is steadily rising, with a 40-fold increase between 1977 and 1995.

The first drug arrest was for possession of marijuana, which had been introduced to the Maldives via a tourist. Then hash and hash oil was introduced. In 1993 brown sugar, a highly adulterated form of heroin suitable for inhaling when heated, but not for injecting, began to enter the country. While expatriates bring it in from its source in Pakistan and Afghanistan via Colombo, these expatriates are not tourists, nor are they linked to the sex trade directly. It is said that the spread of heroin into the islands is facilitated by the safari boats. In some of the capital islands, heroin use appears to be established among young people, but most access is on Male'. When the supply is low on the islands, agents go to Male' for more.

A drug sub-culture has emerged marked by language, clothing styles and probably music preferences. Much of this behaviour is said to be modelled after that seen in films and TV. Clearly, many young people are trying heroin and many are getting addicted, at increasingly younger ages. Drug rehabilitation officers say that the average age of first heroin use is now around 12-14. Examples exist of the recovery of needles from sites of arrest. Drug rehabilitation officers confirm that about five persons have come through their facility who had injected. Presumably they injected the brown sugar heroin or obtained white powder heroin through Bangkok. At the moment injecting is not the main mode of administration.

The spread of injectable buprenorphine use from India/ Pakistan would seem to be a future threat and needs to be monitored carefully. Disposable needles and syringes can be purchased over the counter in pharmacies and the possession of such paraphernalia of drug use would not stand in court alone, but must be accompanied by a drug positive urine test for conviction. Current drug control approaches include a Narcotics Control Board, established in 1997, life (i.e. 25 years) imprisonment for drug dealers and three years imprisonment or institutional rehabilitation for first offenders. Several psychiatrists are associated with the programme at which the addict remains for 4 to 15 months. Presently there are about 120 persons in the programme, nine of whom are female, and there are plans to double its size very soon.

Although there is no detoxification or other biomedical service during which a blood test might be taken, mandatory testing for HIV is planned to begin soon. Some persons, about 20 per cent, have entered the drug rehabilitation facility on their own, without coming through the court system. If an addict is caught by police a second time, there is no chance to return to the rehabilitation programme; they receive a 15 year sentence. As support systems after release are not in place, the relapse rate is estimated to be 70 per cent. Primary prevention to date has consisted of seminars conducted on five atolls to teach parents how to detect if their children are using drugs.

Plans are underway to improve the drug rehabilitation and prevention system, devise a real drug control policy and conduct a rapid assessment of the extent of drug use around the country. Such information and improvement of the programme are sorely needed and should be linked directly to targeted HIV prevention for female users. At present, while HIV is known as a threat by the female users in rehabilitation, they, like other young people in the country, claim they could not use condoms because their boyfriends would feel such use would diminish pleasure.

Condoms are accessible through family planning registration and 36 are given at a time. Registered married couples can access more if travelling. The NGO known as the Society for Health Education (SHE) and government facilities everywhere in the nation, are able to give them free. Accessibility of condoms is not seen by most young people as a major problem as they seem to know condoms can be bought at pharmacies. Many adults do not know this. It is possible that condoms cannot be accessed on some small islands. Condom supply at the medical storerooms in Male' appears sufficient, has standard quality condoms and these are well stored. Shipments are made to the islands every six months, where storage may not be as suitable. UNFPA purchases different brands for the reproductive health programme according to availability and those decisions are made elsewhere. Sometimes a particular brand presents problems and there are complaints.

UNFPA has been responsive to this issue in the past. Use levels appear typically low in the reproductive health programme, with only about 6 per cent of registered couples using condoms. It is possible that the health workers at the end of the chain of distribution are not promoting condom use very strongly, despite the fact that side effects account for the most common reason for discontinuing the use of other contraceptives. In addition, community women seem to worry about the confidentiality of their choice of contraceptives. Family health workers have received information about HIV, but appear to know little about other STDs. Assumptions are made that married couples are generally without need of discussions regarding STDs or protection through condom use. It does not appear that human sexuality education takes place within the reproductive health programme.

All adolescents interviewed in the recent UNFPA reproductive health survey as well as all interviewed for this assessment, knew about condoms for family planning or birth spacing. Several, however, stated that condoms were not trustworthy for avoiding AIDS as they have holes in them. In general, those with higher levels of formal education understand more and this is equally true for males and females.

Female condoms are known by some but there is little experience with them in the country and they are not available at pharmacies. They have a growing acceptance in many areas and have recently been reviewed for re-use, with WHO considering recommending their re-use up to five times with washing. This would bring the price down considerably and make them a real option. Their acceptability in the Maldives might be rather high, as women seem to like to take control of their lives.

BIOLOGICAL FACTORS

Prevalence of Reproductive Tract (RTIs) and Sexually Transmitted Infections (STIs)

The prevalence levels of RTIs in a population can indicate the likelihood of enhanced HIV transmission. For those infections that are sexually transmitted, this information would also provide an estimate of the number of persons exposed through unprotected sex. There is a crossover in this issue because such conditions as bacterial vaginosis, a common RTI, are not sexually transmitted yet are associated with enhanced HIV transmission. As significantly higher prevalence levels can be found by laboratory screening of persons who show no symptoms as well as those who do not recognise the symptoms they do have, only a randomly sampled community-based study can reveal the true levels in a society. No such information is available for the Maldives. All STDs are reportable diseases in the Maldives. As there is considerable fear of being discovered to have an STD, only rare persons would bring STDs to a government facility.

This is especially true in Male' where private health care offers more options. Yet, even private physicians claim that people presenting with STD symptoms always state they did not have sex with anyone but their spouse. Under a legalistic and social system such as that of the Maldives, STD or RTI symptomatic infections are likely to be treated in other ways, or if severe, taken abroad for treatment. In one atoll, people gave the author a local term, kihunu, for a known type of genital discharge in both men and women. Some thought it was equivalent to noria, or gonorrhea. A document from the 1970's states gonorrhea was common in a set of islands and was regularly treated by hakims. In another area the local term of thiyanga bali refers to genital discharge and pain when urinating. The extent of treatment though traditional medicine or over-the-counter drugs or even pharmacist-given prescriptions is not known for the Maldives. Extensive testing for syphilis indicates very low syphilis levels.

Hepatitis B levels appear to be around 6 per cent PID, ectopic pregnancies, cervical cancer and genital discharges are well known to exist. At one Regional Health Centre, there had been 5 PID cases the previous month. RTIs were reported as common on some islands in one large survey of women's health. Informants at IGMH state that ectopic pregnancies seem fairly common. The numbers of cases at government hospitals or clinics can be recovered from in-patient records only. Genital herpes is also known and can be tested for in the country. Levels of resistance of STD pathogens to commonly used drugs is not yet known. Currently syndromic management is being promulgated within the reproductive health programme. Where STDs levels are low, syndromic management is not appropriate for women, leading to a high proportion of overtreatment as well as many missed asymptomatic cases. Given that laboratory facilities are limited and cannot be available at all sites, syndromic management guidelines can be adjusted to fit the epidemiological picture in the community only after a proper STD survey takes place.

Blood-related Transmission

Worldwide, less than 10 per cent of HIV infections have been spread by blood or blood products. In the Maldives, where transfusions are common due to a very high prevalence of thalassaemia, thorough screening of blood donations was instituted early in the HIV control programme. Strong efforts have been made to install universal precautions for infection control in health facilities and these efforts greatly diminish the risk of spread in this manner. Disposable needles and syringes are used throughout the health system. It is clear, however, that although the materials needed, such as latex gloves, are available, not all health workers use them consistently. It is also clear that some laboratory workers are unaware that recapping needles is not recommended in order to avoid needle stick injuries.

The behavioural aspects of infection control among health workers requires repeated inspection and monitoring in order to attain full prevention of the iatrogenic spread of blood-borne infections. The possible exposure of Maldivians to HIV through medical procedures sought elsewhere, as in India, cannot be ruled out. But the number of such cases is likely to be very few and could not alone create the force of infection necessary to sustain an epidemic. Foolhumas (traditional birth attendants) have been advised to use latex gloves.

Some concern has been expressed about the use of razors for men's shaving in commercial salons in Male'. It should be stressed that these and the myriad other possible exposures to blood have no epidemiological importance. While it is technically true that moist infected blood transferred on sharp implements or to the broken skin of a second party in some way can carry HIV, such events are extremely rare and should not be a significant concern of the National HIV Programme. Of course, in public education about the disease it is valuable for people to know that such transmission is possible; it is more valuable for them to know that wiping any surface with bleach that is wet with blood would obviate all risk. Once dried, blood spots cannot sustain live HIV.

The Government of Maldives has shown considerable concern about HIV since the first case was discovered in 1991. Even earlier in 1987 it had established a National AIDS Control Programme. Later a National AIDS Council was formed as a multi-sectoral body with the intention of developing a response across many sectors of society. Day-to-day operations of the programme take place in the Department of Public Health, staffed with a single AIDS Activity Manager and Programme Assistant. During its first years the programme carried out a considerable number of awareness raising activities among seamen, tourist resort workers, secondary school students, health workers, school teachers, religious leaders, and many others. Funds from various donors, including UN agencies, were accessed for both training and specific activities. Surveillance was instituted.

During the past 4-5 years, the momentum has dropped, possibly because surveillance revealed very few cases. Since then, the primary activity has been the continued extensive mandatory testing of an increasingly larger proportion of the population. While it is understandable that some people were alarmed when the first few cases of HIV were found, it is unfortunate that the epidemiological expertise was not available to inform a more useful program effort. Much time and money has been wasted in testing low risk people, in an unsound plan, and not using the available resources for adequate research and prevention.

It is noteworthy that a previous consultant for WHO in 1997 reviewed the system and made very similar comments. Overall, the work accomplished to date has certainly raised awareness of the disease among the nation's people, but it has relied on the fear to accomplish prevention. Throughout the world experience has shown that fear does not motivate lasting behaviour change, although many nations have tried it. To date it appears that HIV prevalence remains very low, despite the proximity of India and its rapidly growing epidemic. This is fortunate and provides an additional window of opportunity for the Government of Maldives to prepare itself and adjust its prevention program in accordance with sound data produced though proper surveillance and research.

Surveillance

The philosophy underlying the present surveillance system is case detection. In many ways, it represents an over-reaction to a few cases found early in the programme. Mandatory screening for HIV began early in 1989. All blood donors were included. At that time WHO recommended screening antenatal clinic patients and sailors. The Maldivian AIDS Council further included all major surgical patients, anyone getting a medical check-up, thalassaemia transfusion recipients, and incoming migrant workers, the latter at their own expense. Because one man with HIV died of TB, TB patients were also included in surveillance. Some people with STDs and domestic maids as well as tourist resort workers have also been tested. A category called 'contacts' was also tested.

In 1995-96 the only unlinked anonymous testing took place as a random one-off sample of various groups. Now students or others who have been abroad for about a year are also tested. Some informants believe students must be tested before acquiring a visa to travel abroad as well. While government facilities test all antenatal patients, ADK states that they only test those who will deliver at their hospital. Seamen are tested after being out at sea for 6 months or more.

Mandatory linked screening, often without informed consent, and always without pretest or post-test counselling continues without change at central and regional hospitals, although the experience worldwide with HIV surveillance since the 1980s has led to alterations in recommended procedures. If pre- and post-test counselling had been done for all the tens of thousands of people who have been tested, how much better HIV prevention would have been served! An enormous opportunity has been missed, which is one of the reasons such testing is not recommended. Although both HIV and other STDs are reportable diseases, the programme does not produce a regular summary report, except recently for counts of those tested monthly and annually and those found positive for HIV. Until 1995, no records were kept or collated on those tested. Some groups are not reported; others are ill-defined.

Surveillance documentation does not provide any information on the socio-demographic characteristics, such as age or sex, of those tested or those tested positive for HIV. No sampling protocols have been made available to participating clinics, although one does exist that suggests inadequate sample sizes and some questionable procedures. In any event, this document is not followed by those participating. Laboratory workers follow the directions in the test kits, mostly several different types of HIV spot tests purchased by WHO. These require linked names as they do not draw enough blood for confirmation; the patient must be called back. This is not a suitable test for surveillance, but may be appropriate for blood donors if Western blot confirmation is skipped and the blood of anyone positive on the first ELISA is rejected. No one should be bled in a linked manner without pre- and post-test counselling. All positives are confirmed at IGMH, the chief government hospital, with a second different ELISA test, followed by a Western blot. In the case of incoming migrant workers, confirmation is not performed and they are simply rejected for a work visa due to health reasons.

HIV testing is not linked in any way to STD screening, risk behavioural surveillance or prevention activities. Because the surveillance is conceived as a net in which to catch or detect positives for the protection of others, the National AIDS Programme in Maldives has limited evidence of the extent of the epidemic in the nation and no way to evaluate the impact of its own activities. With a serious HIV epidemic rising in some parts of neighbouring India and an overall continuing rise in Asia as a whole, the nation of Maldives is obliged to face the great need for improved information. Proper surveillance is the basis of all disease control efforts and, while difficult where diseases are sexually transmitted, is possible in the most unlikely sociopolitical environments wherever public health authorities enlist the political commitment to do so.

The policy statements contained within the Health Master Plan constitute the guidelines for the National AIDS Programme. Some aims have been accomplished, such as widespread awareness raising, thorough blood donor screening, instituting infection control, and some degree of condom distribution, while others have not. Some aims were a bit confused at the time they were written, making execution quite difficult. For example, the document states that testing will be with informed consent but without pretest counselling. Until HIV counsellors were trained, only unlinked anonymous surveillance should have been allowed as proper informed consent is not possible unless a person is given a full understanding of the implications of being tested. This is especially true where treatment is not being offered. Numerous constraints, particularly with regard to trained personnel, have caused a slowdown in activities.

A renewed effort will require a different approach to policy-making. While policy statements have been written that stigma will be reduced, no efforts have been made to bring HIV positive people into the prevention efforts of the country. Older notions that maintaining confidentiality alone will reduce stigma no longer are valid. In many countries, it has been shown that overemphasis on maintaining confidentiality increases stigma. Much of what is done as part of the HIV control programme, particularly in surveillance, contributes directly to the stigmatisation of the disease and the people who may acquire it, though this is not recognised. Considerable fear and denial seems to motivate these activities. As a result, institutions such as one Centre for the Elderly and Disabled, have built special rooms for the isolation of people with HIV.

A serious effort must be made to reverse this trend. Even without exposing the few individuals with HIV in the Maldives, much greater humanisation of people living with HIV/AIDS can be accomplished through the media and in other ways. The policy states that the spread of HIV will be prevented, but methods by which that might be accomplished have never been well-articulated, other than providing safe blood to those in need and creating awareness.

The Maldivian HIV prevention message is seen as a generic one for all, i.e. to maintain mutually faithful monogamous relationships, in spite of an essentially non-monogamous marriage pattern and the clearly recognised reality that unmarried persons engage in sex with presumably several partners before marriage. The promotion of greater fidelity either in marriage or in premarital relationships is possible with carefully designed life skills programmes. Condoms are mentioned as protective, but are not to be promoted. Some young persons appear to have been told that condoms are frequently defective and cannot be trusted. Even AIDS education conducted for seamen does not take up the demonstration and teaching of condom skills. Yet, one very important move has been accomplished with regard to condoms, i.e. making them available at private pharmacies. Several activity reports mention planned research activities, some with regard to behaviour and others on STDs.

There is an over-reliance on fear of detection and arrest to control sexual behaviour. Although legal prosecution for illicit sex is relatively uncommon, informants state that the crowded conditions on Male' lead to numerous disputes amongst neighbours, creating conditions in which people may be turned in to authorities out of vengeance. More women than men are actually punished for illicit sex by the law.

Among sentenced youth, young women predominate over young men, representing 73 per cent (661/902) of non-drug related arrests in 1997. The three main offences for which these persons were arrested were simple theft, illegal coitus and assault/misbehaviour. These figures seem to indicate that sexual offences by females are increasingly attracting the attention of the law. This legalistic approach to sexual behaviour is not likely to improve the situation. The trend since 1990 shows an increasing number of young offenders sentenced by the courts.

UN SUPPORT TO AIDS CONTROL

UN agencies have attempted to coordinate activities with the National AIDS Council. As might be expected, WHO has been the most involved since the mid-1980's. WHO has provided technical support, sent public health staff to meetings and training programmes and funded awareness activities. In addition it has supported the purchase of testing kits for surveillance. As WHO's Global Programme on AIDS turned over to UNAIDS in 1996, funding shifted to WHO's regular programme budget. In 1996 a UN Theme Group was started to unite all UN agencies in an AIDS prevention effort. While some activities did take place, funding and role difficulties thwarted greater action. In 1997 A WHO consultant made a review of the surveillance system. The UN Theme group was re-newed in early 1999 with the inclusion of the Director General of the Ministry of Health and has been the mechanism by which this assessment was formulated and funded. UNFPA has played a role in the leadership of the UN Theme Groups as well as its major role in carrying out reproductive health research and programmes. These activities indirectly support HIV prevention through education and the purchase of condoms.

UNDP has played a leading role for a time in the UN Theme group and funded training as well as the attendance at meetings for health officials. Its role will increase through the support of the development of a drug policy, a rapid assessment of drug use, improved drug abuse treatment and prevention. UNICEF has had no direct AIDS programme, but any work done to improve the position of women, adolescents and children has societal repercussions on HIV prevention.

UNICEF, however, has contributed to the support of the current assessment and is likely to become more involved in the future.

NGOs

NGO development in the Maldives is at an early stage. Their roles, complementary positions vis-a-vis government, funding, staffing and management issues need to be worked out. Nonetheless, expertise and experience within the small NGO sector does exist and must be utilised. SHE conducts a sizable programme on reproductive health, and can refer patients with RTIs to IGMH. Counselling is available from both SHE and Fashan. SHE, Fashan, and KIDS have participated in various ways in awareness building, along with the Department of Public Health. Their involvement in the building of AIDS awareness throughout the country has been recognised and could be expanded.

Monitoring and Evaluation

Evaluations of the different efforts in HIV prevention made so far have not taken place. One might consider the results of the UNFPA reproductive health study as good evidence that a large portion of the population knows something about HIV but little about other STDs, indicating a positive impact on HIV awareness of the total efforts made to date. In the future, proper baseline studies and monitoring is needed to assure that investment is not wasted.

REFERENCES

A Situational Assessment of HIV/AIDS in the Maldives for the Year 2000, UN Theme Group on HIV/AIDS, 2000.

Ministry of Health, Republic of Maldives, Health Master Plan 1996-2005.

Rasheeda A., Maldives Country Paper for 11th Meeting of National AIDS Programme Managers, Jakarta, 1995.

9

Bhutan: Towards a Beginning in AIDS Control

The first case of HIV/AIDS in Bhutan was reported in 1993. Although the first HIV/AIDS was diagnosed in the country in 1993, the testing of army recruits that year did not find any infection in this population group. As of April 2001, 22 persons have been diagnosed with HIV infection, out of which 4 have died. Recent trends show an increase in the number of people diagnosed with HIV/AIDS and as a result, the government has redoubled its efforts for preventing HIV and it's implications to the Bhutanese population. The issue is considered important because the incidence of STI have been quite significant in the past. The current number of HIV estimates is about 100 in 2000.

Compared to other South Asian countries, the prevalence of HIV/AIDS is low in Bhutan, at present. Nevertheless, officials are concerned that even a landlocked country in the remote Himalayas cannot escape from the danger of HIV/AIDS. Bhutan's population of 600,000 are mostly subsistence farmers living in sparsely populated villages across the Himalayas. The literacy rate increased from 23 per cent in 1980 to 54 per cent by 1995, and life expectancy at birth rose from 48.0 to 66.1 years during the decade 1984 to 1994.

The 1994 health survey revealed considerable progress in the health sector, with a dramatic fall in mortality rates. The population is primarily rural, with agriculture as the principal source of income. However, since most arable land is already in use, population pressures and a free inheritance have led to a situation where some households possess insufficient land to meet subsistence needs, fuelling rural-urban migration.

The population of Thimphu, the capital, has been growing at the rate of 10 per cent per annum in recent years. Also the border with India is open with large numbers of people moving freely across in both directions, and a growing number of Bhutanese are travelling abroad.

General health conditions have improved significantly since the 1960s when Bhutan began to modernise. The government has allocated more than 25 per cent of its total budget to the social sector. Health and education are free. Recently, the health services introduced tele-medicine as a cost-effective way of delivering health services to a remote and scattered population. As Bhutan opens up to the rest of the world, HIV could also get a bridgehead in the country.

Nevertheless, HIV/AIDS is on the increase in the country. According to a recent survey, four people with AIDS have died (two men and two women) and 18 people are HIV-positive. Most of them are between the ages of 15 and 35 years. Phuentsholing, a commercial town on the border with India, is the main high-risk area for HIV/AIDS. Many sex workers are active in this town, and an estimated 90 per cent of the town's hotels are involved, directly or indirectly, in prostitution. Health workers target Phuentsholing as one of the areas most prone to sexually transmitted infections (STIs).

Some of the factors that contribute to the spread of HIV in Bhutan are clearly related to development; they include:

i) Bhutan borders India and is located near Nepal, where HIV/AIDS already is an urgent problem
ii) more business people and civil servants are travelling outside the country as Bhutan opens up to global society
iii) increasing rural-to-urban migration
iv) sex work is on the increase

v) low awareness of the implications of unsafe sex
vi) high STI-incidence among certain groups and in certain parts of the country
vii) sexual relations are less restricted compared with other countries in the region
viii) safe sex matters are not discussed at interpersonal level.

NATIONAL RESPONSE

Bhutan's National HIV/STI Control Programme started in 1988 and adopted a multi-sectoral initiative involving all sections of society. The programme is integrated into the decentralised national health system and focuses on HIV prevention. Its activities include condom promotion and free distribution in urban and rural areas through hospitals, basic health units, health workers and private outlets. This has resulted in a higher number of condoms being distributed and used. Education and awareness on HIV/AIDS have been taken to rural communities and information on HIV/AIDS has been inculcated into the education curriculum. The Health Ministry's information education activities maintain a sustained momentum in the awareness campaign.

The country has expressed strong political commitment to fight the spread of the epidemic. Under the guidance of His Majesty, the King Jigme Singye Wangchuck, the government of Bhutan has accorded top priority to HIV/AIDS awareness and prevention activities. Her Majesty the Queen Ashi Sangay Choden Wangchuck, the UNFPA Goodwill Ambassador, has been instrumental in creating greater awareness about HIV/AIDS and reproductive health among all Bhutanese people, especially women and children. With more than 25 per cent of the government's total budget allocated to the social sector, health and education are provided free in Bhutan. The government tries to fulfil the rights of every citizen to good health and full education, leaving no community or section of society unreached.

The government of Bhutan had developed a medium term plan for the prevention and control of STDs and HIV/AIDS in the early 1990s, even before HIV was first diagnosed in the country. Since then activities undertaken have included the establishment of an HIV sentinel surveillance system, the screening of donated blood, the training of health workers at all levels, and the promotion of condom use. STD/AIDS prevention activities have been decentralised and carried out in an integrated manner from the inception of the programme.

In Phuentsholing, a multi-sectoral task force works with commercial sex workers to halt the spread of HIV. Regular STI-treatment campaigns are undertaken, targeting the general population and specific target groups such as sex workers. Currently, activities include promoting HIV/AIDS awareness among the school youth. Information about reproductive health and HIV/AIDS has recently been introduced into the high school curriculum. Community leaders are also becoming involved in awareness programmes in rural areas.

Her Majesty Queen, in her capacity as a UNFPA Goodwill Ambassador, regularly visits different parts of the country to discuss reproductive health issues and HIV/AIDS with women, youth and leaders. Her Majesty plays and instrumental role in creating HIV/AIDS awareness in the country. The commitment on the part of the royal family and government is an unusual and positive factor in the region's response to the HIV/AIDS epidemic. In addition, the Assembly of People's Representatives recently urged government to step up activities to minimise the impact of HIV/AIDS.

The relatively egalitarian gender relations in Bhutanese society are another positive factor. Women's position is strong, particularly at household level, and their negotiating power in sexual matters is relatively good. As Bhutanese attitudes to sex are relatively liberal, HIV prevention programmes are pragmatic and realistic; e.g., condoms are distributed to everyone, including to unmarried people and adolescents.

Serious bottlenecks for effective implementation of the HIV/AIDS programme exist as well, however. Bhutan is heavily dependent on donor funding and may find itself short of funds when it steps up HIV/AIDS activities. Data to support implementation of programmes are available only to a limited extent. Implementation of HIV/AIDS programmes at the community level is often hampered by problems of accessibility.

With high STI rates and the process of opening up to the rest of the world, it is realistic to expect that the HIV rate will increase. At the moment, interventions focus mainly on sex workers. Better scrutiny of who are the most vulnerable groups could enhance the effectiveness of interventions. The increasing numbers of HIV-infected persons will require more resources for counselling. Finally, the country should prepare for the time when the health care system and people at home will have to care for people suffering from AIDS. Other issues such as confidentiality and rights of people with HIV/AIDS also deserve attention. Bhutan could build on experiences and lessons learned in neighbouring countries and adapt them to the local situation.

An in-depth assessment of the at-risk or vulnerable population groups, has been carried out and appropriate awareness and risk reduction interventions are being put in place in pilot areas. Efforts have been made to include HIV/AIDS awareness into the curricula of schools and teacher training institutes, and there have been several initiatives aimed at informing young people in meaningful ways. Other groups targeted for information and education campaigns include transport workers, the army and police, Buddhist monks, and border populations.

UN SUPPORT

WHO, DANIDA, and more recently, UNDP have been assisting the Government of Bhutan in implementing HIV/AIDS prevention and control activities and supporting the surveillance of STDs and HIV/AIDS. UNFPA has been supporting awareness building and education activities, and promotion of condom use, with special focus on high-risk groups such as truck drivers and migrant workers. Special attention is also being given to the reproductive needs of adolescents, as there is increasing evidence of sexually transmitted diseases in this age group. NGO participation is, so far, minimal.

A film featuring the participation of Her Majesty the Queen Ashi Sangay Choden Wangchuk of Bhutan in the 5th ICAAP in Kuala Lumpur and her Keynote Address at the "Satellite Symposium on Socio-Economic Causes and Consequences of HIV and AIDS", has been produced and distributed in Bhutan.

Bhutan has so far had few reported cases of HIV/AIDS. But no nation is immune. And given the prevalence of sexually transmitted diseases in Bhutan, and the alarming HIV/AIDS situation in neighbouring countries, Bhutan is at serious risk. To combat the virus before it becomes widespread, the Royal Government has therefore established taskforces in all districts. UNDP has been supporting the taskforces—building their capacity, helping them access technical assistance and establish policy direction. The taskforces are now drawing up action plans, initiating awareness campaigns, and providing recommendations to the centre.

REFERENCES

Bhutan Ministry of Social Services, Medium Term Plan and Control of AIDS in Bhutan, 1990-1993, WHO Report, 1993.

HIV/AIDS in Asia and the Pacific Region, 2001, WHO Report, 2001.

10

AIDS Vulnerability and Migration Patterns

The spread of HIV/AIDS epidemic is clearly linked to rapid economic transition, such as that being experienced by South Asian countries in the wake of globalisation. Changes such as growing social inequality, rural unemployment, greater poverty, increased mobility, break up of communities, and erosion of traditional values are increasing the vulnerability of large segments of the population of the region to HIV/AIDS. In the last few years South Asia has witnessed a 100 per cent increase in the incidence of HIV infection, and according to UNAIDS, already has over 5 million people living with HIV/AIDS. HIV is primarily affecting the socially and economically productive age group of 15-49, massive numbers of whom are on the move within the region and beyond. These people on the move are broadly described as migrants. They are people who move from one place to another temporarily, seasonally or permanently for a range of voluntary and/or involuntary reasons, including the search for livelihoods.

Migration patterns across South Asia include internal and inter-country mobility, as well as migration to outside the region. The countries of South Asia include sending and receiving countries, as well as transit countries. All these countries are also experiencing large-scale internal migration: migration trends are not only from rural to urban areas but also rural to rural, urban to urban, and urban to suburban. An increased demand for female labour is also leading to an trend of feminisation of migration across the region. A large number of people in the South Asia region are jobless and/or living below the poverty line. Those who are mobile are most often seeking opportunities to improve the living conditions for themselves and for their families. For many individuals and households in the South Asian region, migration has become an important survival strategy. The freedom to move for the enhancement of personal capabilities or livelihood opportunities is therefore an important freedom. So that, HIV/AIDS prevention and intervention strategies need to be directed at reducing the vulnerability of migrants, not at reducing or controlling migration.

Recent analysts of the trends in the South Asia region have recognised that migration generally results from the decision making of collectives such as families or households. The risks associated with migration are therefore backed by the resources of the whole family, in the hope of future benefit to all. The decision is often based on little more than an ill-defined sense that life will offer more elsewhere, with very little information about the reality the migrant will face. According to the International Organisation of Migration (IOM), migration and population mobility are best seen as a process with stages comprising:

i) *Source:* from where people come, why they leave, what relationships they maintain at home while they are away;
ii) *Transit:* the places through which people pass, how they travel, how they maintain themselves while they travel;
iii) *Destination:* where people go, the attitudes of people they meet when they get there, the living and working conditions in the new place;
iv) *Return:* the communities to which people return, their families, their resources.

Most population movements are highly fluid, with people moving back and forth through these stages frequently, often over the course of days, weeks or months, and both within countries and between them. To be effective, HIV/AIDS responses must address the particular needs and vulnerabilities of mobile people at each stage of the mobility process and in a variety of different geographic locations.

The countries of South Asia comprise sending, receiving and transit countries, some of which are both or all three. From most countries of the region, workers are going to the Middle East, and to destinations farther east, including Korea and Malaysia. Within the region, workers from Bangladesh are going to Pakistan and India, between India and Nepal, there is movement in both directions, as well as between Sri Lanka and the southern states of India. The Maldives receives large numbers of migrant workers, especially in the tourism industry. Within the countries of the region, rural-urban movement is increasing rapidly, and the established patterns of seasonal migration of farm labourers are becoming increasingly complex with changes in agricultural practices and productivity.

Migration trends in the region depend largely on socioeconomic factors as well as the past migration experience of the source community. The movements also rely on the availability of local livelihood options and proximity to metropolitan cities. An analysis in Nepal, for example, has identified various categories of migrants, in which destination of migration is linked to socioeconomic conditions, education status, access to information and existing networks as well as the extent to which the migrant can harness resources to fund the migration. Across the region statistics for migration give a partial estimation of the scale of the movement of populations, based on official figures for recorded departures of migrant workers. These do not reflect the complex informal and undocumented migratory movements which are also taking place.

Internal migration is omitted or poorly reflected in most census and sample surveys, although several countries in the region have taken steps to amend this in recent survey rounds. As for the relationship between migration and HIV vulnerability, though research has been limited to date, preliminary studies indicate direct linkages between migration and HIV vulnerability. According to figures from the Bureau of Manpower and Employment and Training (BMET) of Bangladesh, the average number of documented migrant workers, both skilled and unskilled is about 200,000 per year. There is very little documentation of internal migrants, but the major cities have huge slums housing individuals from throughout the country as well as the region. The constant flooding of different parts of the country also lead to frequent population displacement. The UNAIDS estimated HIV prevalence in Bangladesh in 2000 was 21,000. 41 per cent of the detected cases are in migrant workers. This could be because this is the group most systematically tested.

According to the National Sample Survey in India (1993), 24.68 per cent of the population, or approximately 200 million people, were recorded as having migrated, either within India, to neighbouring countries or overseas. Recent studies have estimated the annual flow of workers overseas to be well over 100,000 people, 80 per cent from the unskilled sector. An estimated 1.5 million Indians are in the Middle East. India also receives many migrants. It is estimated that anywhere between 1.8 and 3 million people from Nepal alone come to India for their livelihoods. In terms of HIV infection, India has one of the largest populations of people living with HIV/AIDS in any country. Recent UNAIDS estimates suggest that 3.86 million people are living with HIV/AIDS in the country.

The Nepal Department of Labour has registered 52,170 overseas migrants since 1989, but this figure does not include the vast numbers of people crossing the open border into India on a daily, weekly and monthly basis. Within Nepal, there is a constant flow of movement from the hills to the plains in search of work. Reports of villages where there are no resident males of working age are further indications of this trend. Over 18,000 people have been detected as HIV-positive, but it is estimated that there are more than 80,000 already infected. Drug use and migration are considered to be among the key factors contributing to the spread.

Figures provided by the Bureau of Emigration and Overseas Employment of Pakistan for 1999 record 2,790,221 nationals working abroad. Within the country's borders, all major cities host migrant populations from both within Pakistan and outside, and over a million Afghan refugees remained in Pakistan as of the end of 2000. Roughly 20 per cent of the population of Karachi consists of individuals who have come from other provinces or are migrants from various countries. According to UNAIDS, reported HIV cases in 1999 were 74,000. Out of a sample of 9000 individuals from high-risk groups who were tested for HIV in Karachi, 85 per cent were positive. Of these, 44 per cent were overseas workers, 8 per cent were the spouses and children of overseas workers, and 9.3 per cent were frequent travellers.

According to a 1999 report of the Government of Sri Lanka, 178,000 people are reported to have left Sri Lanka for employment abroad that year. The total number of Sri Lankans abroad is estimated to be around 788,000 of whom 90 per cent are in the Middle East, Saudi Arabia, Kuwait and the United Arab Emirates. Of these, approximately 66 per cent are housemaids. Sri Lanka has been identified as a low prevalence country for HIV, with only 7,500 in 1999, according to UNAIDS. However, more than 65 per cent of cases detected are said to have a connection to a foreign sexual contact. Further, among the females deemed positive, 50 per cent are migrant workers. This could merely reflect the systematic testing of this group.

Migration is a reality for many individuals working or in search of work within the region. Due to economic hardships, lack of economic opportunities as well as exploitation and harassment, many migrant workers are faced with very harsh realities. The country reports in this publication describe these hardships and the difficult experiences faced by those who leave their homes in search of work. The majority are poor, do not have access to health services, and are exploited and neglected. Foreign workers may not be covered by the same legal protections as their national counterparts, and they are generally unaware of their rights as workers. Moreover, they have unstable lifestyles as they have insecurity in their jobs, are culturally alienated from the place where they work, and often lack access to social support systems. It is these very challenges that make these individuals more vulnerable to HIV infection.

HIV VULNERABILITY AND MIGRANT WORKERS

Migrant workers are not an economic tool or commodity in the international labour markets, though they are often treated as such. Many migrants work in low paid, unskilled jobs, in hostile environments. Their vulnerability to HIV arises largely from their human need for company, intimacy, and sex.

Workers who are new to an area, either from a different part of the country or from another country altogether, are often already marginalised throughout the process of getting to their new place of work. Their differences, including language and cultural background, often subject them to alienation, discrimination, exploitation, and harassment. These individuals have little or no legal or social protection in their host community. These factors increase their vulnerability to HIV infection as well as to the difficulties of living with HIV/AIDS. Being away from their families, their home communities, and familiar sociocultural norms can lead to isolation and loneliness, often exacerbated by discrimination.

In some cases, the disconnection and alienation, as well as exhaustion and pain caused by dirty, dangerous and demeaning work (3D work) can lead migrant workers to turn to substances for solace. Reports from drug treatment centres have shown high numbers of migrant workers seeking treatment, indicating that migrant workers can be at risk of substance use and abuse, including injecting drugs. This in turn leads to higher risk of HIV exposure. Vulnerability also arises from the social and economic conditions in which people live and work. These include the uncertainty about their employment and even their legal status. In India for example, 92 per cent of workers are in the informal sector, largely unprotected by laws or unions, and the majority of these are migrants. The majority of migrant workers are placed in unskilled jobs and illiteracy is common.

Being in unfamiliar territory, Migrant groups often have poor living and working conditions. They may also ignorant of the services available to them, as well as often being unfamiliar with the social norms prevailing in their host country. Given their lack of awareness, these migrant workers have little access to HIV information, health services, testing and treatment centres for sexually transmitted infections and means for HIV prevention. Cultural and linguistic barriers heighten their lack of access to the services that exist. They might not even know where or how to obtain a condom, even if available. Women migrants are particularly vulnerable, and many face sexual exploitation and abuse from employers, middlemen, or even other migrants. The low socioeconomic status of women in society across the region is exacerbated by being away from home and from familiar systems of social protection. Many are deceived by traffickers who promise good jobs, only finding out that they have been trafficked once it is too late. Much trafficking of women and children is disguised as recruitment to the international labour markets. Well-intentioned attempts by governments to protect women by limiting or banning their migration through legal channels, ironically only heightens their vulnerability to trafficking, as women who seek to migrate are thus forced to move through illegal channels and to depend on dubious middlemen.

Migrant workers, especially those who have moved through illegal or unofficial channels, or have had their documents taken away from them by employers or others, may avoid attention from authorities, even if that attention is meant to provide health services, or to help improve their living conditions. They may also be uncomfortable or inexperienced in relating to the non-governmental or community-based organisations that may be in place to help them, and thus not approach them for assistance. Poverty and lack of resources may force those moving from one place to another to increase their risk of HIV by trading or selling unprotected sex for goods, services and cash in order to survive and/or continue their travel. In some countries, they may also face the possibility of being tested for HIV against their wishes or without their knowledge. Their HIV status may be revealed to authorities in their destination or source countries, or to their communities and families. Such breaches of confidentiality give rise to stigma, discrimination and rejection. On the other hand, deportation without being advised of HIV status, leads to anger, confusion and vulnerability of sexual partners.

Generally, migrants and mobile people are exposed to unique pressures, constraints, and living environments. Many are separated from their families and spouses or regular partners. They may feel anonymous, or they may also feel freed from the social norms that guided their behaviour in their home family, community and culture. Their loneliness may provoke some to engage in behaviours they would not have otherwise. In some settings, living and recreational environments for migrants and mobile workers are almost exclusively male.

Coupled with attitudes relating to appropriate male behaviour and peer pressure this can lead to the development of commercial sex services and the pressure to use them. It may also lead to increased sex among men. Further, it may also increase the use and abuse of illegal substances including alcohol and drugs, which in turn increase vulnerability and susceptibility to HIV infection. For those workers who have left partners at their source community, visits home can become the means by which HIV infection is brought to otherwise unexposed communities. In many remote and rural areas in Asia and elsewhere, HIV incidence can often be directly linked to migration.

Vulnerability of migrants starts in the source community itself, where the decision to migrate is often guided by desperation, an absence of choices, misinformation and often unrealistic expectations. Generally, literacy levels are low and access to information to guide decision-making about migration, as well as information on HIV/AIDS, is very limited. The countries in the South Asian region have large percentages of their populations living in poverty with very few employment options. They are deeply affected by the rapid economic transition taking place within the region. People are exposed to growing social inequality, rural unemployment and poverty and break down of their communities and traditional value systems. Their state of anxiety and hopelessness makes them desperate for alternative options.

Migrants returning to their homeland are often unaware of whether they have been exposed to HIV and of the potential risk to their spouse and unborn children. Those returning because of illness due to various opportunistic infections in most cases are not aware that HIV is the cause of their poor health, and many are deported without explanation if tested HIV positive.

In the current climate of stigma and discrimination and absence of treatment, those who know that they are HIV positive rarely feel empowered to share this knowledge or to protect their partner or spouse. Most source communities therefore are not aware of the relation between HIV and the migratory process, or how migrants can protect themselves from infection. Some communities in Nepal, once made aware through the insertion of HIV messages into poverty alleviation programmes, have started letter-writing campaigns to their members who have migrated sharing the information with them.

Besides the vulnerability of migrants themselves, spouses left behind may also be at risk of unprotected sex with other partners. Women who occupy a very low status in society are at risk of sexual exploitation, particularly when debts have been incurred by the migration and remittances fail to come. Girl children may be at an increased risk of sexual exploitation and exposure to traffickers recruiting for the sex industry in the region. The lack of involvement of migrant returnees, spouses of migrants as well as migrant source communities overall in national HIV prevention responses adds to the vulnerability of migrant workers and their families.

In Sri Lanka the government has recently expanded its pre-departure programmes for migrant workers to the community in a phased manner. The information on safe migration, HIV, and other issues is disseminated through innovative methods, to target children, adolescents, youth and the older population. In Bangladesh work in this direction is being carried out by various civil society organisations, offering some models for the region. This kind of information can be especially useful to potential female migrants, especially young women. Family pressure can play an especially significant role in women's migration decisions.

A study in Bangladesh has shown that families tend to urge women to migrate where they are perceived as a burden to the family, or are seen as of potential economic benefit. Through migration they can be instrumental in sharing the family's economic burden, including earning for the education of male members of the household. This is especially true because women are seen to be more reliable at sending back remittances than their male counterparts. At the same time, for some women, migration can provide an escape route from limitations imposed by traditional societies, and abuse or violence at home Thus the facilitation of safe migration can be viewed as a strategy for women to gain control over their lives. Initiatives within source communities can inform and empower all groups of migrants, including those who will move within the country and those who will go farther, and can also be influential in preventing trafficking.

The factors that pertain vulnerability to HIV are related to the migratory process from the source community to the destination. In the case of overseas migration the lack of formal training, law enforcement or regulation of recruitment agencies and the system of middlemen make many migrants easy prey to fraud and exploitation. Where rigid emigration laws are imposed, both for migrants going overseas and internally within in the region, unregulated migration through informal channels flourishes. These migrants are at higher risk of being cheated and exploited as well as facing dangers *en route*, and in particular women become vulnerable to sexual harassment, exploitation and trafficking during the course of migration. For people on the move within the region the whole transit environment can be characterised as risky. Prevalence of HIV along the main transport routes has been reported as high, and migrants pass through junctions where commercial sex work and MSM behaviour are common. Being in a state of excitement, stress or anxiety with a little bit of money in the pocket can lead to having casual sex or being lured into substance use.

Routes of migration also often follow the routes of organised crime such as trafficking of drugs, illegal goods, and women and children. Women who start out as hopeful migrants without sufficient information, guidance or protective systems can find themselves trafficked into different kinds of bonded labour, including sex work, within or outside the region. Even women, who start out as legitimate migrants with documents and promises of jobs, may find themselves cheated or sold along the way where effective and powerful traffickers operate. What happens to these women does not remove the legitimacy of their desire to exercise the freedom of mobility in search of livelihood opportunities, but only illustrates the urgent need for measures guaranteeing their safer migration.

In South Asian countries, presently, few effective responses to the needs of people who have taken the decision to migrate have been implemented. Sri Lanka is in the forefront with pre-departure training programmes, regulation of recruitment agencies, insurance and some support to migrants overseas. Over 41,000 unskilled female workers received pre-departure training in the year 2000. In other countries of the region the momentum to address trafficking has led to a number of recent initiatives, but much remains to be done in a concerted manner to mitigate the vulnerability of people on the move within the region and to outside.

Migrant labour is generally treated as an economic commodity by authorities, employers and the general public, with little provision for their human needs. Studies have revealed that the first contact migrants make in the destination area are crucial for their long-term social well being. This is important to keep in mind if migrants are to be empowered to protect themselves, their sex partners and their families from HIV infection. However, in many cases they are met with hostility and marginalisation.

Migrants tend to be considered outsiders by local populations and poor people in the destination areas often see them as competitors for scarce livelihood resources. Lacking access to proper housing, they stay overcrowded slums with no proper facilities and are exposed to hazardous working environments. The vulnerability derived from the general lack of access to health care and other public goods is worsened by racial and cultural discrimination. The general experience is that when they arrive at overseas destinations they are abandoned by the recruiters, and the contracts that were presented to them prior to departure are changed or violated, against which they have no protection.

There are many reports of migrant workers not being paid at all, and of others who are sent to detention centres for illegal migrants after removal of their papers by employers or others. While in many destination countries, as well as in export processing zones within the region, organisation of labour is banned, trade unions within the region traditionally have not addressed migrant workers as part of their mandate. Against this background, disillusionment, insecurity and despair can make people vulnerable to increased risk behaviours, including unprotected sex and drug use. Community outreach work in

Delhi has experienced that about two thirds of the injecting drug users have come from outside the city. Many came to seek work and commenced drug taking after migration. Loneliness, the disappearance of social control, peer pressure, lack of recreational outlets and normal sexual needs of young women and men who lack knowledge of sexual health or protection combine to make them vulnerable to HIV. In the Sri Lankan free trade zones studies have estimated the abortion rate to be 1-2 per cent—a very significant indicator of unprotected sex. The non-availability of condoms and the criminal implications of being found with condoms, especially for women, aggravate the situation in many destination sites.

Women migrants, both in situations of prostitution as well as otherwise, are often victims of violence and harassment. Reports of sexual assault by employers and others are not uncommon both within the region from overseas and legal redress is rarely an option. Furthermore, family pressure for remittances and salaries far lower than promised can lead to supplementation of earnings through sex work, particularly where there is high demand from male migrants. In all these situations the negotiation power of the women for safer sex is extremely low even if they are aware that they might be exposed to HIV.

State of Indian Migrants

India has had a long history of migration, starting when the British moved parts of the population to Sri Lanka, Malaya and other countries to work in developing plantations. Much of the migration in recent years has been a direct result of the prevailing idea that jobs abroad are more lucrative than those found within the borders of India. Despite the enormous support that migrant workers provide to the economy, bureaucratic red tape in processing documents for would-be migrants has spurred the proliferation of illegal agencies who get the job done faster. This leads to the exploitation of people wishing to migrate, both financially as well as physically. Also, often due to a lack of awareness accompanied by misleading employment agencies, many migrants are given false or inappropriate visas for employment, which can lead to them being classified as illegal migrants in the receiving country. The following problems have been identified by migrant workers and organisations working with them:

i) They are often exploited by the agents from the time of getting the passport till leaving the country at every level: it is the middleman [broker] who plays a major role.
ii) Most of the service workers pledge their jewels or dispose of their property to pay huge sum demanded by the agents.
iii) Many migrants are cheated by the agents by being given a menial job in the place of the promised one.
iv) There are also cases in which the migrant worker receives much lower salary than what is promised before departure by the agent.
v) Domestics face sexual abuse in the host country as a result they are not in a position to return as they fear social boycott by the family and the community.
vi) There are cases in which the migrants are given severe punishments with shocking cruelty. There are several cases in which the migrant worker either has died or missing.
vii) Many migrant workers become undocumented workers and thereby lose their status of 'equality before law' because they are sent by the agents on either tourist visa or social visit visa.

Employers have been known to change or violate agreements, underpay or not pay their employees, provide unhealthy working and living conditions, demand long working hours and expose their employees to unnecessary risks. Many migrant workers report being subjected to physical. sexual and psychological abuse, and occasionally, are also subjected to cruel, inhuman or degrading treatment. Sometimes, their identity documents, residence and work permits are confiscated or destroyed. They often do not have equality with nationals of the state before the courts and tribunals. The police and immigration authorities arrest, detain and sometimes summarily deport them without due process. There are also reported cases of physical and psychological suffering by migrant workers in the custody of immigration authorities.

A major trend in the migration patterns of India is the high degree of cross-border migration between India and neighbouring countries. It has been estimated that there are anywhere between 1.8 million and 3 million Nepalese migrant workers in India and conversely an estimated 800,000 to 3.2 million Indians in Nepal. While the majority of these come and go voluntarily, there are also reports of coerced migration and trafficking. For example child-workers from Bihar have been taken illegally by private contractors to build roads in Nepal, and trafficking of Nepalese women and girls as sex workers to Mumbai and other destinations is taking place. As well as weaknesses in the support given to migrant workers who are leaving India for work abroad, there is also little support for those individuals who come to India for work.

These conditions of exploitation make it very difficult for migrant workers to protect their health. The casualisation and feminisation of migration has brought untold misery in terms of health of the workers. The violation of human rights takes place from the day a migrant worker decides to go abroad. They are kept in the capitals or in big cities for months before they leave for the host country as their agents keep them in the waiting, supposedly, to prepare papers etc. This time of waiting, confusion, and sudden removal from the familiar home environment can lead to exposure to HIV. Men usually get their exposure to red-light areas during this period, and women migrant workers are often exploited at this stage. The transit stage is an important stage during the migration process where often the rights of migrants are blatantly violated by recruiting agents and other intermediaries, setting aside the health of the migrant workers. The case of Indonesian women migrants who are housed during transit in overcrowded agency houses marked by sub human living conditions in Jakarta for extended periods of time, often up to a year, is a classic example where no/ poor access to sanitation, nutrition, access to medical care as well as the threat of rape and sexual abuse impacts the health and HIV vulnerability of migrants in transit. The practice of confining prospective migrants to long periods of stay in 'hostels' also takes place in Cambodia.

In India it is in Bombay where the migrants are kept in almost slave like conditions while they await employment in the Gulf countries. Undocumented migrants, especially women migrants who are without legal identities, are more vulnerable to abuse by corrupt and fraudulent recruiting agents, enforcement officials and others at borders who wield much power over migrants. Looking at the transit stage of migrants it is clear that many of the violations of their human rights contributing to their HIV vulnerability arises from irregular migration and of irregularities in the migration process.

Many receiving countries require potential migrant workers to undergo mandatory tests for HIV and other infectious diseases. The question of mandatory testing on migrants for HIV raises many concerns. The first is at the level of the migrant workers' rights. The second is with regard to issues involved in using mandatory HIV testing on migrants as a strategy to manage the HIV epidemic. To assess the logic and ethics of mandatory HIV testing of migrants as a strategy to manage the HIV epidemic we need to look at two other issues—of notification and deportation of HIV positive migrant workers.

For migrant workers, mandatory HIV testing and deportation brings more anger than anything else, especially because of the manner in which it is done. An HIV positive result means that the migrant stands to lose their livelihood. This is everything to people who have been forced out from their land and country by poverty, often after selling or mortgaging their small piece of land or cattle for a job which they thought would help their family and loved ones escape from and hunger and destitution. If they have tested HIV positive but not been informed about the result, or have been informed wrongly or improperly, the human and financial cost and pain for them and their families when they return home is immeasurable. Mandatory testing is not fair either to migrant workers or to the host population in receiving countries. It gives a false sense of security to the local population in the receiving country who think that they are free from HIV because of the mandatory testing and deportation of migrants with HIV. Research and experience clearly indicate that the migration experience puts migrants at the risk of acquiring HIV.

In the issue of mandatory HIV testing and deportation, the rights of migrant workers are violated and include the right to equality and non-discrimination, the right to health, right to social security, right to work and right to freedom of movement. It also isolates them and reduces their participation in fighting the AIDS epidemic. The host country health care system should take responsibility for the health of the migrant workers. In the receiving countries the migrant workers must also be included in national health/HIV information campaigns.

State of Pakistani Migrants

In developing countries, the economic disparity has proven to be a major factor to encourage the movement of people from places with limited opportunities to those with greater opportunities. Other migratory movements such as refugee movement or internal displacement, are often the outcome of political instability and environmental degradation. The causative factors in the case of Pakistan are at times interwoven. In the year 2000, Pakistan had an estimated population of 138 million. In 25 years, it is estimated that the population will double, increasing the strain on infrastructure and resources. The level of unemployment is expected to increase even more in the coming years.

The high rate of population growth, accelerating unemployment rate, and economic conditions in the context of globalisation make leaving Pakistan a viable and often preferable option for many people. Shifting patterns of employment in many Gulf countries as well as the South Asian region are leading to the replacement of unskilled migrant workers with skilled labour. At the same time, many countries are in the process of formulating and introducing policies that reduce the number of migrant workers on the whole. These countries are now faced with the complexity of dealing with those workers who are either illegally employed or are employed on a contract basis. The reduced demand for unskilled labour and consequent competition by recruitment agents undercutting wages sought, make migrant workers even more vulnerable.

The Pakistani migrant workforce is facing serious hardships abroad. Returnees report discrimination of different forms and at different levels, exploitation because of lack of awareness about rights, and alienation because of lack of knowledge about avenues of assistance. In addition, the type of work in which Pakistani migrant workers are involved provides them very little protection. They are largely illiterate and are non-skilled, working as labourers, home workers and in factories. Many times, their subordinate position leads to their exploitation. The lack of the required legal structures and the loopholes in the available structures often lead to the laws being easily flouted.

Pakistan, being both a recipient and a sending country, needs to reappraise and re-evaluate existing policies, legal structures and implementation mechanisms. At the same time as citizens are leaving the country's borders in search of work, citizens from other countries are entering Pakistan with the same objectives, as well as to seek refuge from difficult situations in their own countries. Unfortunately, no data has been collected on these people entering the country, both because no system for data collection has been developed, but more importantly, because many enter the country without documentation. The undocumented migrant workforce is not registered or in touch with any official government channels in order for their numbers to be recorded, and apart from that, they try to remain inconspicuous in fear of being found out and deported. This means that they do not attempt to access even the services that exist or seek redress for exploitation, heightening their vulnerability in many ways, including to HIV.

In Pakistan internal migration has also increased, which is posing new types of challenges because of its repercussions on the socioeconomic spheres. Policies and strategies are required which can deal effectively with the negative impact of the unrecorded internal migration. According to a rough estimate, more than 20 per cent of the population of Karachi comprises those who have either come in to work from other provinces or those who are migrants from Afghanistan, Bangladesh, Burma, Philippines and the Central Asian States. This has an impact on the weak domestic economy and also challenges the social structures of the society.

In order to analyse the demographic impact and the social change of internal and international migration on a developing state like Pakistan it is necessary to measure its influence on the resident population as well as the migrants themselves. Lack of data on internal migration and the illegal workforce has created difficulties in identifying and measuring the challenges posed. A recent survey conducted in the rural areas of Pakistan shows that the majority of migrants leaving rural areas or leaving Pakistan altogether, are male. Leaving the responsibility of agriculture to women who are untrained and unskilled has resulted in a decline in agricultural productivity. It has also changed the gender division of labour on farms.

Vast majority of migrant workers are unskilled and uneducated and employed for manual work, including for jobs such as factory workers, taxi drivers and domestic staff. Even if they possess some basic literacy skills, by and large their level of education and awareness is low. This leaves them open to the risk of contracting infections and being carriers of certain inherent and endemic diseases without any possibility of seeking medical recourse to prevent the risk of spreading those diseases both locally and regionally. The risk factor therefore is maximised by their lack of awareness and failure to consider the health aspect seriously.

In the case of HIV/AIDS, for example, many may dismiss their risk of contracting the infection without a true understanding of the actual risk and vulnerability they may face. Many diseases are particular to certain geographical regions within Pakistan. Poor water supply, nutritional deficiencies, climatic conditions and other such factors may be the reason for such poor health outcomes. As a result, migrant workers may be in poor health at the start of the migration process. It is therefore essential to include in the proposed pre-departure, post-arrival and reintegration programmes a substantial section on health, education and creating awareness amongst migrant workers about various risks and aspects of health.

High stress and lack of avenues for mental support have caused a substantial number of migrant workers to turn to drugs for temporary relief. The most obvious danger of such addictions or even occasional use of drugs is the physical and mental dependency on the substance used. Additional side effects include a loss of appetite resulting in weight loss, decreased concentration and lethargy. From the financial point of view, a continuous use of drugs burdens the already scarce resources, and in turn, this adds to stress levels.

Migrant workers using drugs are therefore caught in a cyclical state of mental anxiety and pressure, which can increase their vulnerability to high risk behaviours. Those who are using injecting drugs are clearly at an even higher risk of vulnerability to HIV infection. Apart from drug use amongst migrant workers, sexual behaviour is also a contributing risk factor. Most migrant workers are single men and most belong to a healthy and reasonably young age group. They do not travel with their families, and are away from home for a long time as travel is an unaffordable luxury, and leaving for a short period may even cost them their job. In the case of illegal migrants the option of visiting home does not exist and they usually leave once they decide to end their stay as a migrant worker, or are deported. In these cases, the duration of time away from their families can be years, and even decades. These workers are often lonely and in the absence of their spouses or being bachelors, many seek sexual fulfilment, including visiting brothels.

The migrant workers often live in cramped quarters, share limited living space with workers from similar backgrounds who are of the same sex. As a result of loneliness, alienation and the close quarters living conditions, sexual relations between men take place. The main attraction of this is the fact that this sexual relief comes for free compared to that offered by brothels and professional sex workers. In all of the above scenarios, the use of protection during casual sex is rare if not absent altogether.

Lack of education, the impulsive nature of the sexual encounters and the cost and perhaps embarrassment of purchasing contraceptive devices are the major contributing factors to this decision. The cost of this unprotected sex increases the chances of contracting sexually transmitted diseases, which include HIV and AIDS. To add a more serious twist to the prevalent scenario, it is speculated that many of the high-risk migrant workers, return to their place of origin being unaware carriers of viruses and diseases. There is no infrastructure for checks on their health when they return, even for migrants who return and leave through legal channels. These situation create a very high risk of the spread of diseases including HIV/AIDS, and make spouses and families vulnerable also.

State of Bangladeshi Migrants

Although a significant number of Bangladeshi workers are migrating every year, and their earnings are a vital contributory fact to the national income, they are facing enormous problems in many ways. Among them is HIV/AIDS. Migrant workers have very little access to information regarding AIDS, and all of them go through mandatory HIV testing without either counselling or confidentiality. Moreover, most migrant workers are not informed of their HIV-positive status if that is the cause of their deportation from their host country.

There are few data on HIV in Bangladesh. However, it is known that the majority of people identified as positive are migrant workers or their spouses. It is possible to identify them, however, because they have mandatory testing before departing from the country. Below is a table of the known occupations of those deemed positive thus far. Without orientation, information or training, young migrant workers often engage in casual or commercial sexual relations to mitigate loneliness and also due to peer pressure. At the same time, Bangladesh on the whole has a lower HIV prevalence. Because there is job scarcity in the unskilled labour force, Bangladeshis should work to maintain a healthy workforce and low HIV prevalence.

To further advocate for programmes aimed at keeping HIV prevalence levels low, it is useful to consider the government recommendations towards more effective STD/AIDS programmes. In the Bangladesh National policy on HIV/AIDS & STD- related issues, it is clearly stated that:

> Peer education and peer outreach works best for certain communities. Strategically located drop-in centres that provide STD services, information and counselling services for vulnerable sectors of society should be strongly considered. These services should be accessible, convenient and sensitive to the needs and particular requirements of the particular targeted group.
>
> For those emigrating for work outside the country, we need to provide education and counselling in places of recruitment. Advocacy work targeted at relevant agencies

> (such as the Ministry of Manpower) towards adoption of policies and regulations favouring the provision of an educational package such as "Health Maintenance Behaviours During Travel" that includes STD/AIDS education, for people leaving to work abroad must be explored. We should also explore networking between NGOs and relevant manpower recruitment agencies.

There are several strategic points where migrant workers can be reached with education and information campaigns before their departure. Stakeholders that need to get more greatly involved include recruiting agencies, medical check-up centres, Bureau of Manpower Employment and Training (BMET), middlemen or the local representatives of the recruiting agencies in each community. So far, very few initiatives respond to the issues faced by migrant workers. SHISUK has been working with the Bangladeshi Overseas Migrant Workers Association on a "Migration and HIV/AIDS" project since 1995.

With the support of the national AIDS programme, UNDP, IOM, HASAB, CARAM-Asia and others, SHISUK has been conducting interventions on information outflow, documentation, media campaigns, policy advocacy, counselling, pre-departure orientation programmes, mobilisation of spouse groups, and a peer educators' programme Shikkha Shastha Unnayan Karzakram (SHISUK's), programmes are focused on meeting the following objectives:

i) Developing and strengthening the migrant voice in advocacy;
ii) Ensuring safe migration;
iii) Ensuring that the rights of migrant workers are respected, protected and fulfilled;
iv) Ensuring safety and security of migrants workers' spouses and family members;
v) Support and strengthen the right to stay as well as reintegration of migrant workers back into Bangladesh;

vi) Ensure the success of the national AIDS prevention, care and support programme. Though SHISUK has been actively involved in responding to the needs and problems of migrant workers, clearly the government and others within civil society need to take a greater role.

State of Sri Lankan Migrants

Migrant workers from Sri Lanka, who are predominantly women. The Sri Lankan Bureau for Foreign Employment (SLBFE) regulates foreign employment, including the licensing and monitoring of recruiting agencies. The Government of Sri Lanka also has arrangements with its embassies in 12 receiving countries to register contracts of Sri Lankan workers. The most recent estimate for the total number of Sri Lankan workers abroad is estimated to be around 788,000 of whom 90 per cent are employed in the Middle East. Saudi Arabia, Kuwait and United Arab Emirates are the principal countries that attract workers from Sri Lanka. The majority of job opportunities made available to Sri Lankans fall into the category of unskilled labour, which includes housemaids. Housemaids account for 49 per cent of total placements in 1999. In fact, the majority of placements in 1999 (65 per cent) consisted of female workers.

The remittances of migrant workers have become the highest net foreign exchange earning source for Sri Lanka. The country earned Rs. 54.9 billion during the period from January to July 1997, which was an 11 per cent increase compared to the same period of the previous year. This is an increase of Rs. 8.4 billion over the earnings by migrant workers in 1996, which amounted to Rs.46.5 billion, constituting 21 per cent of the total export earnings of the country and 7 per cent of GNP. Sri Lankan migrant workers earned Rs. 74 billion in foreign exchange in 1999 and Rs. 84 billion in 2000. Clearly, the government has a keen interest in promoting foreign employment, especially in light of its ever-weakening economy.

The past years have seen an unusual trend towards female migration, with married women outnumbering unmarried

11

AIDS: The Vicious Cycle

According to current records, about 11.8 million young people aged 15-24 are living with HIV/AIDS. Many are vulnerable to HIV because of risky sexual behaviour or substance use, because they lack access to HIV information and prevention services, or for a host of social and economic reasons. Stigma can be particularly damaging to youngsters at a time when they are trying to consolidate their identity and establish their place in the world. Yet, it is also young people who offer the greatest hope for changing the course of the HIV/AIDS epidemic, if they are given the tools and support to do so.

About half of all new adult infections around 6000 daily are occurring among young people. While it is difficult for many adults to admit it, large numbers of young people begin sexual activity at a relatively early age, are sexually active before marriage, are not monogamous, and do not use condoms regularly enough to ensure protection.

In many countries, a significant proportion of young people start sexual activity before the age of 15, and many of them are already married. In addition, experimentation with drug use, including injecting, is often a feature of youth. This underscores the capital importance of implementing prevention programmes long before sexual or drug-injecting activity might commence, because too many young people are unaware of the threat posed by HIV. Marginalised young people are at particular risk if they are excluded from health services, exposed to unprotected sex or use illicit drugs.

The estimated 1 million children who are forced into the sex trade every year are especially susceptible to contracting, and then spreading, HIV/AIDS. In most societies, dominant ideologies promote sexual ignorance among young women. Young people's vulnerability is compounded by their scant knowledge of how HIV is spread and how infection can be avoided.

Many millions still have not heard of HIV or AIDS; many more harbour misconceptions about the disease. In addition, young women in many countries are far less knowledgeable about HIV than are young men. Half of the teenage girls in sub-Saharan Africa, for example, do not realize that a healthy-looking person can be HIV-positive. But even where knowledge has been substantially increased, 'knowing' is not necessarily 'doing'. Many young people do not connect knowledge and risk perception with behaviour.

The vulnerable circumstances many young people experience might offer a partial explanation. Just as important is the need to understand what helps young people practise safe behaviour — the protective factors that help adolescents form coping strategies, develop positive self-esteem and create a social support system that reduces high-risk behaviours.

One study in rural Zimbabwe, for example, demonstrated that being a member of a well-run community youth group can reduce a young woman's chance of becoming infected with HIV. A 2001 study among South African students suggested that condom use is significantly greater among adolescents who feel they can discuss sex with their parents, or adolescents who live in communities with good infrastructure. In contrast, young people living in households that recently experienced disruptive household events were less likely to use condoms.

The future course of the epidemic depends on the efforts mounted today to prevent HIV infection among young people. Taking as an overall principle the conviction that young people are themselves a force for change, several basic strategies are essential to helping young people protect themselves. These include:

i) protecting and promoting the rights of the child, including the rights to information, education, health and health care, freedom from rape and sexual coercion and cruel and inhuman treatment, and the right of girls to equality in education, employment, inheritance, marital law, and sexual and reproductive decision-making;

ii) providing HIV/STI prevention, sexual and reproductive health and life-skills education and information to young people, whether they are in school or not;

iii) providing reproductive health services, including low-cost or free condoms, voluntary counselling and testing, and diagnosis and treatment of sexually transmitted infections;

iv) targeting programming to particularly vulnerable groups such as young injecting drug users and young men who have sex with men; and combating sexual exploitation of young people.

These strategies are most effective when they take into account the role of gender inequalities in the epidemic, and when they help empower girls and young women against a wide variety of cultural and social inequities that make them more vulnerable than males.

Despite the obvious threat to young people's health and lives, HIV/AIDS is still too frequently regarded as an 'unsuitable' issue for them. But prevention programmes for young people in school are an essential component of any national HIV prevention effort. Several important lessons have been learned about how to do this effectively. Programming should be sustained, starting before puberty and continuing throughout a young person's school years.

Many authorities resist the idea that such education should begin before young people become sexually active. But the timing of people's sexual debuts varies widely, and the importance of good health habits, including those regarding sexual health and HIV/AIDS and other sexually transmitted infections, must be driven home at an early age. Preventive health education should be comprehensive, providing an age-appropriate balance of life-skills development, reproductive and sexual health information, and discussion of attitudes and values.

The more information provided, the better, according to a recent study that compared teenage sexual and reproductive behaviour in high-income countries. Relatively low rates of teenage pregnancy and sexually transmitted infections in countries such as Canada, France and Sweden seemed to reflect the success of comprehensive curricula, applied on a national scale, covering a wide range of topics and presenting options for safe sexual behaviour. Less successful outcomes were reported in school systems where abstinence was presented as the only appropriate option for teenagers outside of marriage, and where contraception was incorrectly presented as ineffective in preventing pregnancy, HIV and other sexually transmitted infections.

Other common features characterize successful programmes. Among them is the consistency of messages: successful curricula provide and reinforce clear messages about the risks of teenage sexual activity, and how to either avoid intercourse or guard against pregnancy and sexually transmitted infections. Adequately trained teachers who support the programmes increase the potency of such programmes. These programmes also need to take account of traditional beliefs and value systems, as well as the popular mythologies that circulate among young people and their wider communities.

The value of promoting safer sex through education and communication campaigns risks being lost if young people do not have access to further information, advice and reproductive health services, and to treatment for sexually transmitted infections. In many high-prevalence countries, such services are scarce and, even if they exist, young people do not know about them. Current best practice in youth-friendly health services shows they should be affordable, cater to minors or unmarried adults, and offer low-cost or free condoms in an atmosphere that guarantees confidentiality. And, in many settings, flexible opening hours for young people who work or study will make a big difference to the number of people who use such services.

More targeted HIV prevention programmes are needed for specific groups of young people. For example, young men who have sex with men, or who are unsure about their sexuality, may be reluctant to access services geared towards the heterosexual majority. In many countries, the majority of sex workers and injecting drug users are young people. And in all countries, the majority of sex workers and injecting drug users start these activities when they are young. With more and more young people turning to injecting drug use in many countries, there is a growing need for preventive programmes specifically adapted for young injecting drug users. These include substance use and drug rehabilitation services, as well as needle-exchange programmes and education on HIV prevention. The same is true for young sex workers. Given the hazards they face, they need more information, regular health check-ups, and easier access to condoms. Just as importantly, they need support and protection to use these services. Specially-designed programmes can be useful in reaching young people who are already in the workforce.

Young people who have had trouble with the law and are living in detention centres or jails are especially vulnerable. Recently, UNFPA worked with Thai health authorities and non-governmental organizations to bring HIV/AIDS education to juvenile delinquents living in a detention centre in Rayong Province. The project took the innovative approach of involving family relations of the detained young people, and study tours outside the centres.

One of the most pressing challenges is to halt the widespread sexual exploitation of young people and children, especially young girls. This priority received powerful support in December 2001 at the 2nd World Congress against Commercial Sexual Exploitation of Children in Yokohama, Japan. The Congress presented a wealth of evidence of the dangers to which children are subjected, and underlined the connection to HIV/AIDS. The meeting's final declaration the Yokohama Global Commitment provided a broad framework for fighting this exploitation.

Children trapped in prostitution are at higher risk of infection, being both less able to resist sexual dominance and more vulnerable to the injuries of aggression. Children's subservient role in commercial sex means that they are often obliged to take multiple clients each day. Solutions must necessarily be multi-sectoral, with law-makers and law-enforcement organizations playing a large part. Efforts to change cultural attitudes through mass media campaigns also have an undoubted role.

IMPACTS OF HIV/AIDS

In many countries, AIDS is erasing decades of progress made in extending life expectancies. Average life expectancy in sub-Saharan Africa is now 47 years, when it would have been 62 years without AIDS. Life expectancy at birth in Botswana has dropped to a level not seen in that country since before 1950. In other African countries, life expectancy has dropped less severely, but it is still significantly below what it would have been without AIDS. The impact of AIDS on life expectancy, which signifies a major blow to a society's development, has spread beyond Africa. Haiti's life expectancy in 2000-2005 is nearly six years less than it would have been in the absence of AIDS. In Asia, Cambodia has experienced a reduction of four years. Current HIV prevalence levels merely hint at the much greater lifetime probability of becoming infected with HIV.

Even relatively low prevalence today can mean high odds of contracting HIV. In Guyana, where adult prevalence is 1998, the probability of contracting HIV between the ages of 15 and 50 in 2000–2035 is 19 per cent.

High as they are, these estimates are conservative, and assume that HIV infection rates will decline in the future, as stronger prevention efforts bear fruit. In the 45 most affected countries, it is projected that, between 2000 and 2020,68 million people will die earlier than they would have in the absence of AIDS. These projections are based on the assumption that prevention, treatment and care programmes will have a modest effect on the growth and impact of the epidemic in most countries over the next two decades. The assumptions do not include a reduction in the annual number of newly infected people, which would result from vaccination with a possible future vaccine or from use of other possible future technological advances. Nor do they include the potential effect of large-scale future access to antiretroviral therapy on the survival of people living with HIV/AIDS. The projected toll is greatest in sub-Saharan Africa, where 55 million additional deaths can be expected 39 per cent more deaths than would be expected in the absence of AIDS. AIDS has a particularly strong impact on mortality among children between the ages of one and five. Most children who are infected at birth or through breast-feeding will develop AIDS and die before their fifth birthday. In the worst affected countries, HIV/AIDS has had a major impact on child survival. In seven countries in sub-Saharan Africa, under-five mortality has increased by 20–40% due to HIV/AIDS.

The toll of HIV/AIDS on households can be very severe. In many cases, the presence of AIDS means that the household will dissolve, as parents die and children are sent to relatives for care and upbringing. A study in Zambia revealed that 65 per cent of households in which the mother had died had dissolved. But much happens to a family before this dissolution occurs; HIV/AIDS strips the family of assets and income-earners, further impoverishing those already poor.

In Zambia, AIDS has led to a rapid transition from relative wealth to relative poverty in many households. Research shows that, in two-thirds of families where the father had died, monthly disposable income fell by more than 80 per cent. This was often the result not only of the loss of income due to illness among household members, but also because other members had to divert more time and effort away from income-generating activities. A study of three countries has calculated that AIDS will not only reverse efforts to reduce poverty, but will increase the percentage of people living in extreme poverty from 45 per cent in 2000 to 51 per cent in 2015. In Botswana, per capita household income for the poorest quarter of households is expected to fall by 13 per cent, while every income-earner in this category can expect to take on four more dependents as a result of HIV/AIDS. Loss of income, additional care related expenses, the reduced ability of care givers to work, and mounting medical fees and funeral expenses collectively push affected households deeper into poverty.

Studies in Thailand and the United Republic of Tanzania show that the financial burden of death can be far greater than that of illness. Households there have reported spending up to 50 per cent more on funerals than on medical care. Traditions in many societies require that relatives and community members gather (sometimes for several days) at the home of the deceased to mourn and support the bereaved. In many cases, lengthy journeys are required to reach a burial place. Three main coping strategies appear to be adopted among affected households. Savings are used up or assets sold; assistance is received from other households; and the composition of households tends to change, with fewer adults of prime working age in the households. Tapping into savings and taking on more debt are usually the first recourse by households that struggle to pay for medical treatment or funeral costs.

In an ongoing study in the Free State Province of South Africa, households used up, on average, 21 months of savings to pay for medical expenses and funerals. In the United Republic of Tanzania, a case study has revealed that, in households where one person was ill because of AIDS, 29 per cent of savings were redirected to cope with the illness. As debts mount, precious assets, such as bicycles, livestock and even land, are sold. Once households are stripped of their productive assets, the odds of them recovering and rebuilding their livelihoods grow ever slimmer.

Thailand, revealed that 41 per cent of AIDS affected house holds reported having sold land, 57 per cent used up their savings and 24 per cent had borrowed from a cooperative or other type of locally run fund. In response, many households restructure themselves: dependent children might be sent to live with relatives, or relatives may join the household to assist in household or farming tasks. One of the more unfortunate responses to a prime age adult death in poorer households is that of removing the children (especially girls) from schools as school uniforms and fees become unaffordable and the girls 'labour and income generating potential are required in the household. Almost invariably, the burden of coping rests on women as the demands for their income-earning labour, household work, childcare and care of the sick multiply. As men fall ill, women often step into their roles outside the homes; in parts of Zimbabwe, women are moving into the traditionally male-dominated carpentry industry, for example.

HIV/AIDS poses a potentially major threat to food security and nutrition, mainly by diminishing the availability of food (due to falling production, and loss of family labour, land, livestock and other assets) and reducing access to food as households have less money. Research in the United Republic of Tanzania has shown that individuals 'food consumption dropped by 15 per cent in the poorest households after the death of an adult. The prospect of widespread food shortages and hunger is real. Some 20 per cent of rural families in Burkina Faso are estimated to have reduced their agricultural work or even abandoned their farms because of AIDS. In Ethiopia, AIDS-affected households were found to spend between 11.6 and 16.4 hours per week performing agricultural work, compared with a mean of 33.6 hours for non-AIDS-affected households. With fewer people available to work in the fields, households often farm smaller plots of land or switch to less labour intensive subsistence crops, which often have lower nutritional and/or market value. Although yields drop and incomes shrink, farming households may still cope, especially in areas where different crops can be planted throughout the year. Where one or two key crops must be planted and harvested at specific times of the year, however, losing even a few workers at the crucial planting and harvesting stages can scuttle production. These kinds of difficulties are being experienced also in countries with lower national HIV prevalence rates and, in early 2002, they prompted the United Nations World Food Programme to coordinate a food donation scheme for families affected by HIV/AIDS in four Asian countries (Cambodia, China, Laos and Myanmar). A similar plan was being proposed for southern Africa. The World Food Programme has also run food security projects for women widowed as a result of AIDS.

Since nutrition requires an integrated approach to household food security, health and care, it forms a logical entry point for helping affected communities to cope with the epidemic. Securing the right of women and children to retain the land and assets of a deceased husband/father, for example, helps households cope. Other remedies include promoting less labour intensive crops that still serve as nutritious food sources, and setting up or expanding school based feeding programmes. For example, UNICEF is extending the role of schools as community resource centres an initiative that complements the World Food Programmes' proposal that school-based feeding programmes include 'take-home rations'.

Impact on the Health Sector

In all affected countries, the HIV/AIDS epidemic is bringing additional pressure to bear on the health sector. In countries where per capita health expenditure is low, extending prevention and care for sexually transmitted infections, counselling and testing, prevention of mother-to-child transmission services; and HIV treatment and care strains health budgets and systems. As the epidemic matures, the demand for care of those living with HIV/AIDS rises, as does the toll taken among health workers. In sub-Saharan Africa, the annual direct medical costs of AIDS (excluding antiretroviral therapy) have been estimated at about US$30 per capita, at a time when overall public health spending is less than US$10 for most African countries. Even in high-income countries that appear to be holding the epidemic at bay, the pressure on health budgets and health insurance schemes is significant. At the turn of the century, the direct medical costs of treating HIV/AIDS patients in the European Union ranged from about US$3400 per person annually, in the early stages of symptomatic HIV infection, to more than US$50 000 in the latter stages of AIDS.

Health-care services face different levels of strain, depending on the number of people who seek services, the nature of the demands for health care, and the capacity to deliver that care. In the early stages, HIV infected persons (often experiencing common bacterial infections) tend to use primary health care and outpatient services. As HIV infection progresses to AIDS, there is an increase in total hospitalisations related to HIV/AIDS. The 2001 Swaziland Human Development Report estimated that people living with HIV/AIDS occupied half the beds in some health care centres in that country.

HIV prevalence among hospitalised patients was almost 33 per cent in one Tanzanian hospital, making HIV infection the major cause of illness leading to hospitalisation. In Zimbabwe, 50 per cent of all inpatients in wards studied were infected with HIV. Without major interventions, the problem will worsen. The World Bank estimates that the number of hospital beds needed for AIDS patients could exceed the total number of beds available in Swaziland by 2004 and in Namibia by 2005.

Hospital occupancy rates, though, can underestimate the impact on health services, since hospitals in some areas might already be operating above capacity. Several studies have suggested that the epidemic is having a negative impact on the overall quality of care provided. A shortage of beds, for example, means that people tend to be admitted only at the later stages of illness, reducing their chances of recovery, as some Kenyan hospitals have discovered. Lengthy hospital stays are being reported in Botswana's hospitals, meanwhile, along with staff shortages and staff burnout. Up to 30 per cent more time is being spent diagnosing and investigating cases that have grown more complex as the epidemic intensifies.

Demands for counselling have increased, while hospital expenses on drugs, linen, blood, and HIV and other tests have risen by up to 40 per cent. Beyond the increased burden on hospitals and health care facilities, there will be a significant increase in costs for basic health care as the epidemic expands. At the same time, the demand for health services is expanding and more health-care personnel are being affected by HIV/AIDS. Malawi and Zambia, for example, are experiencing 5 -6-fold increases in health-worker illness and death rates. To compensate, the training of doctors and nurses would have to increase by an estimated 25–40 per cent in 2001–2010 in southern Africa, for example. Increased workloads and stress might also spur emigration by health professionals.

Recognising the need to but tress the health sector, African leaders attending the Organisation of Africa Unity's special summit on AIDS in April 2001 pledged to allocate 15 per cent of their total annual budgets to health care. The emergence of community rooted home care initiatives, often organised by people living with HIV/AIDS, have become one of the outstanding features of the epidemic and a key coping mechanism for mitigating impact. Although initiated by communities and often operating from a religious or non-governmental organisation base, the effectiveness of home based care depends on support from formal health, welfare and other social sectors. A recent exercise calculating the likely cost of providing home-based care and support countrywide in South Africa concluded that, while not cheap, it is an affordable option.

Impact on the Education Sector

The extent to which schools and other education institutions are able to continue functioning will influence how well societies eventually recover from the epidemic. A decline in school enrolment is one of the most visible effects of the epidemic, the contributing factors include: the removal of children from school to care for parents and family members; an inability to afford school fees and other expenses; AIDS related infertility and a decline in birth rate, leading to fewer children; and the fact that more children are themselves infected and do not survive through the years of schooling.

According to research by the Health Economics and AIDS Research Division of the University of Natal in South Africa, for example, the number of pupils enrolling in the first year of primary school in 2001 in parts of KwaZulu Natal Province was 20 per cent lower than in 1998. Economic hardship was a major factor in this reversal, but the study also suggests that some children were not living long enough to enter school. In the Central African Republic and Swaziland, school enrolment is reported to have fallen by 20–36 per cent due to AIDS and orphanhood, with girls most affected. AIDS is also hampering the ability of education systems to perform their basic social mandates, as more teachers succumb to the disease.

A recent study in Manicaland, Zimbabwe, found that 19 per cent of male teachers and almost 29 per cent of female teachers were infected with HIV -almost exactly the same proportion as among working men and women in the general population. According to the South African Democratic Teachers Union, nationwide AIDS-related deaths among teachers rose by over 40 per cent in 2000 -2001, as calculated from claims to the union's funeral plan between June 2000 and May 2001. Illness or death of teachers is especially devastating in rural areas, where schools often depend heavily on one or two teachers. Moreover, skilled teachers are not easily replaced. Swaziland has estimated that it will have to train 13 000 teachers over the next 17 years just to keep services at their 1997 levels -7000 more than it would have to train if there were no AIDS deaths. While the loss of teachers and administrators directly affects the quality of education, there is also the danger that demands on the health and welfare services might divert resources from education to other sectors. The costs associated with training new teachers and hiring substitute teachers will also strain budgets, crowding out investments in infrastructure, materials and human resources. Such improvements are especially necessary for countries aiming to compete in an increasingly knowledge-based world economy.

Among the efforts to avert such outcomes is the World Bank's Ed-SIDA Initiative. Along with creating tools for proactive planning and management, the scheme trains education planners to model changes in the supply of, and demand for, education. Examples include making projections of teacher illness and mortality, calculating whether there will be sufficient teachers to meet education goals, and analysing the changing realities and needs of students. To date, planners from 10 African countries have participated in Ed-SIDA training, and the Initiative is being extended into other countries in sub-Saharan Africa. Impact on enterprises and workplaces HIV/AIDS dramatically affects labour, setting back economic activity and social progress.

The vast majority of people living with HIV/AIDS worldwide are between the ages of 15 and 49 in the prime of their working lives. Productivity and profitability are core concerns for enterprises, large and small. AIDS weakens economic activity by squeezing productivity, adding costs, diverting productive resources, and depleting skills. In addition, as the impact on households grows more severe, market demand for products and services can shrink. The epidemic hits productivity mainly through increased absenteeism, organisational disruption, and the loss of skills and 'organisational memory'. Rising absenteeism tends to push visible costs up while forcing productivity down, putting profits at risk. Production cycles can be disrupted, equipment stands idle and temporary staff may need to be recruited and trained. Comparative studies of East African businesses have shown that absenteeism can account for as much as 25–54 per cent of company costs. Quality control of products and services often suffers, which can erode the customer base. A study in several southern African countries has estimated that the combined impact of AIDS related absenteeism, productivity declines, health care expenditures, and recruitment and training expenses could cut profits by at least 6 – 8 per cent. Nam Water, Namibia's largest water purification company, has reported that HIV/ AIDS was hindering its operation as absenteeism rose and productivity rates dropped.

The impact on informal enterprises can be especially harsh. When the lead entrepreneur is no longer able to work, there is a high risk that the entire enterprise will collapse. High rates of absenteeism, morbidity and mortality trigger increasing disorganisation in workforces, as a result of rising staff turnover, loss of skills, and weakened morale. A study of a bus company in Zimbabwe showed that AIDS-related absenteeism accounted for 54 per cent of all AIDS-related costs, followed by HIV-related symptomatic illness at 35 per cent. Loss of know-how tends to be the most often-cited cost factor on the shop floor. Thus, even in high unemployment areas, the drain on visible and invisible skills and knowledge ends up being considerable. To respond to these problems, companies must invest in increased training and recruitment. Company costs for health care, funeral benefits and pension fund commitments are likely to rise unexpectedly as early retirements and deaths mount. A study of a commercial agricultural estate in Kenya showed that AIDS related medical expenditure surpassed projected expenses by 400 per cent.

Funeral costs are also provided by a number of employers, especially in Africa, and these are rising sharply. However, these effects are not confined to countries of the South. In the United States of America, the Centers for Disease Control and Prevention has reported that firms with around 1000 employees found that the five-year cost to their business ranged from US$17 000 to US$32 000 for each worker with HIV. Supporting prevention programmes therefore makes good economic sense. Health care provision is also a good investment since it limits or prevents sickness and absenteeism.

Many enterprises still do not regard the epidemic as a major threat. Rapid assessments carried out by ILO in enterprises of various sizes and sectors surveyed managers' perceptions of the epidemic. In South Africa, while more than 60 per cent saw the epidemic as a very serious threat at national level, only about 20 per cent thought it seriously threatened their enterprises. Of those employers alert to the problem, most said it already affected productivity and the effects were visibly increasing costs. Although enterprises in trade and finance reported little visible impact on their health bills, most said they were affected by increased absenteeism.

Macro-economic Impact

Through its impact on the labour force, households and enterprises, HIV/AIDS can act as a significant brake on economic growth and development. Reliable knowledge of the impact of HIV/AIDS on the national economy and its various sectors and participants is valuable for effective national strategic planning and necessary for strong advocacy. A range of studies agrees that the net effect of the epidemic on per capita gross domestic product (GDP) growth is negative and possibly substantial. For those countries with national HIV/AIDS prevalence rates of 20 per cent, annual GDP growth has been estimated to drop by an average of 2.6 percentage points. More recent calculations have suggested that the rate of economic

growth has fallen by 2 –4 per cent in sub-Saharan Africa as a result of AIDS. Meanwhile, nationally focused studies have forecast that, by 2015, the economies of Botswana and Swaziland would grow by 2.5 and 1.1 percentage points less, respectively, than they would have in the absence of the epidemic. Long term scenarios developed for Mozambique indicate that AIDS would reduce gross domestic product and could discourage foreign and domestic investors. By the beginning of the next decade, South Africa, which represents about 40 per cent of sub-Saharan Africa's economic output, faces a real gross domestic product 17 per cent lower than it would have been without AIDS. One study has forecast that South Africa's economy would grow 0.3 – 0.4 per cent less annually in 2000 – 2015, than it would have in the absence of the AIDS epidemic. Research has also shown that, despite the fact that AIDS would have the most impact on relatively unskilled sections of the labour market, unemployment levels would remain largely unchanged.

According to an annual investor survey by Business Map SA, the AIDS epidemic has increased the risk profile for investment in southern Africa. Investors now seek premium rates of return of 15 – 20 per cent in South Africa and an even higher 25 per cent or more in the rest of the region. The economic impact is forecast to hit home on other continents, too. Research at the University of the West Indies has estimated that AIDS could cause an average 5 per cent loss of GDP by 2005 in Jamaica and Trinidad and Tobago. One study has projected that gross domestic product in 2005 would be around 4.2 per cent lower in the Caribbean than it would have been in the absence of the epidemic.

More research is required to achieve greater precision in the modelling of macro-economic impact. It is particularly important to distinguish the impact of AIDS on weakening economies from other negative factors such as declining terms of trade, heavy debt burdens and the effects of structural adjustment, weak governance systems, political instability and conflict. Per capita calculations can also disguise and underestimate the human impact of AIDS. The epidemic kills people, as well as eroding economic productivity. In settings where informal economic activities feature strongly, measured economic output only scratches the surface of the total impact of HIV/AIDS on livelihoods, food security, community welfare and the destinies of societies.

Security at Risk

AIDS generates more demand for resources and services at all levels of society, while simultaneously weakening the underpinnings of the economy and the State. On the economic and development fronts, several of the worst-affected countries were already struggling with daunting development challenges, excessive debt burdens and declining terms of trade before the epidemic hit. This is most obvious in many sub-Saharan African countries, but is increasingly becoming the case in some countries of the former Soviet Union where socioeconomic setbacks have accompanied economic restructuring. HIV/AIDS is exacerbating these frailties in numerous ways. If effective responses are not introduced and the epidemic is allowed to grow unchecked, its multiple effects could cascade across society, heightening the risk of insecurity, as policy-makers are now beginning to discover. Recognising the security implications of HIV/AIDS. The UN Security Council made history in January 2000, when, for the first time, it debated a health issue. By subsequently adopting Resolution 1308 (2000), it highlighted the potential threat the epidemic poses for international security, particularly in conflict and peacekeeping settings.

The AIDS epidemic weakens many of these pillars of social cohesion. This is because HIV/AIDS, along with other factors (such as conflict and economic stagnation), can have a destructive effect on human security (i.e., on people's right to safety from the threats of hunger, disease and repression). This is especially important in light of the fact that many countries in both the region with the fastest growing epidemic (Eastern Europe) and the region with the highest national HIV prevalence rates (sub-Saharan Africa) are fledgling democracies, where restructured State bureaucracies are trying to foster the trust of citizens. In many of the countries worst affected by HIV/AIDS, States' capacities to support households have suffered in the past two decades. By adding further pressure to national budgets and by weakening State institutions, the epidemic makes it even more difficult for the State to perform one of its primary duties: protecting citizens from human suffering, including hunger, disease and destitution.

The epidemic does not spare the educated and skilled personnel who administrate and manage State and other large institutions. In Zambia, nearly two-thirds of deaths among managers have been found to be attributable to AIDS, while an ING Barings study has forecast that 23 per cent of South Africa's skilled workforce will be HIV-positive by 2005. As the provision of essential services falters (most obviously in health, education, welfare and justice) the poor and most vulnerable households endure the worst of the consequences. Even where traditional or new, locally-based social safety nets manage to hold, the failure of the State to adequately support these community-driven coping systems can dent its legitimacy.

The epidemic's potential impact on the rule of law is especially important. Although statistics are hard to come by, attrition rates among staff serving in law and order institutions in high prevalence countries appear to be on par with those in other sectors. In Kenya, for example, it is estimated that AIDS accounts for up to three quarters of all deaths in the police force. The sector also includes judges, prosecutors, court clerks and lawyers all players in maintaining the rule of law and sociopolitical stability.

A State less able to provide social services may unwittingly foster political alienation and weaken its own political legitimacy. Through its impact on both State and community capacity, AIDS can thus contribute to social disruption and perhaps even civil unrest. Such disruption invariably hurts the most vulnerable sections of society. Children orphaned as a result of AIDS, for example, are left especially vulnerable in such circumstances and, in some settings, can be lured into military/paramilitary activities with the prospect of 'family' bonds and the promise of food and consumer commodities.

STRATEGIC PREVENTION

The global HIV/AIDS epidemic is made up of many different epidemics that are evolving in tandem, often within the same country. Effective HIV prevention combines society-wide strategies with particular focus on those parts of the population most at risk. Whatever the extent of the spread of the epidemic, young people need to be at the centre of all HIV strategies not least because most HIV infections occur during, or soon after, adolescence. Strategies that work combine:

i) AIDS life-skills education;
ii) mass media communication;
iii) access to condoms;
iv) voluntary counselling, testing and referral;
v) treatment of sexually transmitted infections;
vi) involvement of parents and other adults; and
vii) efforts to improve young people's social and economic status.

In low-prevalence settings, a concentrated epidemic tends initially to be associated with certain high-risk contexts typically, sex work, injecting drug users and sex between men. Usually, these activities are also highly stigmatised. But the people at risk in these contexts are not isolated groups; they mix across populations, as confirmed by behavioural surveillance.

However, early, large-scale interventions among these groups could stave off a potential epidemic. In high-prevalence settings, the epidemic is spread much more broadly throughout the general population. The higher the national HIV prevalence rate, the higher the proportion of people who must adopt safer behaviour if the epidemic is to be brought under control. Very high coverage with demonstrably effective interventions then becomes crucial. Whether in low-or high-prevalence areas, the key to effective prevention is to apply essential prevention strategies to the realities of the epidemic, at the local, national or even regional levels.

Twenty years into the HIV/AIDS epidemic, the majority of countries in the world still register national HIV prevalence rates of less than 1 per cent, for the global epidemic is still in its early stages. But two decades ago, there was no country in the world that had nationwide adult HIV prevalence rates above 1 per cent; today there are nearly 50 and, in 12 of them, national adult HIV prevalence is estimated to be more than 10 per cent. HIV rates, as a national average, can be misleading. In populous countries, national adult HIV prevalence of, say, 2-3 per cent may nevertheless mean millions of infections. National HIV prevalence rates can also mask the concentrated nature of HIV epidemics in specific parts of the country and among specific populations. Large-scale epidemics always begin as localised outbreaks before spreading more widely across regions and communities. In Nairobi, Kenya, HIV prevalence among female sex workers surged from 4 per cent in 1981 to 61 per cent in 1985, while prevalence among pregnant women rose from 0 per cent in 1981 to only 2 per cent in 1985, before its subsequent steep rise.

The danger signs of impending epidemics are now familiar, but the exact pace of the epidemic's growth still cannot be predicted with certainty. In Thailand, for example, the virus was first detected in 1984, but did not start spreading virulently among sex workers and their clients until five years later. Similarly, in the Nepalese city of Kathmandu, needle sharing was rife in the early 1990s, yet HIV infections among injecting drug users stayed negligible for six or seven years before rising sharply to the point where, by 1997, nearly half the users were infected. In Indonesia, anonymous HIV testing of sex workers began in 1988 and, for almost a decade, registered virtually no HIV infection. The results were puzzling because other research was showing that sex work was common, condom use very low, and other sexually transmitted infections highly prevalent. The absence of a HIV epidemic may have been partly because sex workers in Indonesia had a relatively low turnover of partners around seven in a week, on average, compared with over 30 a week in Thailand at the height of the HIV rise in that country. But new data suggest that there has been a surge in HIV infection among sex workers in some Indonesian locations. Large-scale migration, in the wake of the 1997–98 economic crisis and political instability and violence in parts of the country, may also explain increased vulnerability.

Prevention and Condoms

Condoms are key to preventing the spread of HIV/AIDS and sexually transmitted infections, together with sexual abstinence, postponement of sexual debut, and mutual fidelity. Uganda's success in curtailing the spread of HIV can be attributed to behavioural change, notably a reduction in the number of individuals' sexual partners and the postponement of sexual debut among young people. Decline in infection rates among young people has been mostly due to the rise in the median age of first intercourse by 2 years-from age 15 to 17. But increased condom use and treatment of sexually transmitted infections have played an important role. The US National Institutes of Health and the US Centres for Disease Control and Prevention conducted an extensive review of available studies, and confirmed that condoms, when used correctly, are an effective means of preventing HIV infection in women and men, and gonorrhoea in men. Without access to condoms, many other prevention strategies lose much of their potential effectiveness.

An estimated 6–9 billion condoms are distributed annually (including those sold commercially)— considerably fewer than the estimated 8–24 billion condoms that are needed if all populations are to be able to protect themselves from HIV and other sexually transmitted infections. In sub-Saharan Africa alone, the condom gap has been estimated at 2 billion a year. To overcome the supply gap, the United Nations (through the United Nations Population Fund, World Health Organisation and the UNAIDS Secretariat) is collaborating with international non-governmental organisations, specialised agencies and public and private donors. Cost is a major issue. The United Nations Population Fund estimates that the number of condoms needed to prevent HIV/ AIDS and other sexually transmitted infections will more than double in the next 15 years. Costs will rise from US $239 million in 2000 to an estimated US $239 million in 2015. This total does not include distribution, training or counselling costs. Low-income countries will need plans that address supply problems along with steady increases in donor support to meet condom costs. Increasing condom accessibility and availability can increase condom use. In Brazil, there was a massive increase in the uptake of condoms when prices came down in the early 1990s. When Ford South Africa made mass condom distribution part of its HIV/AIDS strategy and put condom distribution machines in work place toilets, uptake increased 25-fold.

However, supply is not the only determinant of condom use. Almost everywhere, sexually active young people are denied information about condoms. Researchers in Kenya report that 54 per cent of young people do not believe that condoms protect against HIV infection. There, as in many other countries, attempts by government and non-governmental organisations to promote condom use have met with opposition from some religious organisations that claim that condoms promote promiscuity.

But religious opinion is not monolithic. In Uganda, for example, a dialogue between the Islamic Medical Association and Muslim religious authorities resulted in a statement by the latter that education an the responsible use of condoms was both acceptable within Islamic teachings and necessary to defend communities against AIDS. A recent analysis of study samples from eight countries in sub-Saharan Africa found that attitudes towards condom use also depended on the nature of relationships. In marital and regular relationships, many people said that they did not use condoms because they 'trusted' their partner; in regular and casual relationships, people frequently cited a dislike of condoms. This suggests that condom promotion messages need to be tailored to context: couples in steady relationships may need to be convinced that using condoms is a primary means of caring for each other's health.

Condom programming works best as part of a comprehensive package of interventions that include HIV/AIDS education, sexual health and human sexuality, and gender sensitivity training. Since it was first introduced by public health authorities in Ratchaburi Province, Thailand's innovative 100 per cent Condom Use Programme for commercial sex has become known as one of the most effective HIV prevention measures ever. The programme required that condoms be used in all sex work establishments a tactic that helped prevent clients moving on to locations where condom use was not insisted on. After being adopted as a national policy by the Prime Minister in 1991, and expanded nationwide, the programme resulted in more than 90 per cent of sexual encounters with sex workers by 1994 being protected by condoms.

The programme worked with sex workers and their clients, health authorities and the police, and gained brothel owners support. At the same time, the Thai Government embarked on large-scale, mass-media, AIDS-awareness campaigns. Recent reviews of the programme credit it with being an important contributor to large-scale reduction of HIV transmission throughout the country. Social marketing the use of commercial techniques such as market research, mass-market distribution and communication to achieve a social goal has achieved some success. In Cambodia, condom social marketing has been promoted since 1994. Number One brand condoms are marketed to young adults, commercial sex workers and their clients, and members of the military and police. Sales of condoms in Cambodia increased dramatically from 99 000 to more than 16 million in 2001, with distribution to all 24 provinces and municipalities. These types of interventions, though, need to be buttressed by policies that ideally promote, but, at the very least, do not restrict, the distribution and use of condoms. Unfortunately, laws and practices in many countries still make it difficult for young people to get condoms, and allow the possession of condoms to be used as evidence to prosecute sex workers.

Controlling Sexually Transmitted Infections

The World Health Organisation estimates that over 300 million people are infected each year with curable sexually transmitted infections, a large share of which occur among young people. The presence of such infections magnifies the risk of HIV transmission during unprotected sex as much as tenfold. Many of these infections can be cured relatively easily with antibiotic treatment. But lack of services, poor availability of drugs, limited access to diagnosis, and disparaging attitudes by service providers are barriers to more effective detection and treatment of sexually transmitted infections as part of HIV/AIDS prevention. These problems are surmountable. A great deal has been learned about making services more user friendly, and adapting them to suit specific groups. In addition, research in low and middle income countries has confirmed the effectiveness of syndromic management in resource poor settings. Syndromic management involves recognising clinical signs and patient symptoms and prescribing treatment for the major causes of that syndrome. It enables health workers who lack specialised skills and access to sophisticated laboratory tests to effectively treat most symptomatic infections during a patient's first clinic visit.

Several recent studies highlight the likely importance of the Herpes Simplex Virus-2 (HSV-2) as a co-factor of HIV susceptibility. A study in South Africa has found that HSV-2 was the most significant factor associated with HIV among both men and women, and that men infected with HSV-2 were seven times more likely to be HIV-positive than those without it. HSV-2's co-occurrence with HIV indicates that HSV-2 control (both prevention and treatment) may be a valuable part of HIV prevention.

Treatment for the ulcers requires relatively expensive drugs, only one of which (acyclovir) is available in generic form. Moreover, testing for HSV-2 is difficult in poorer countries, because affordable testing kits are not as accurate as the laboratory-based tests used in wealthier countries. In such conditions, early sexual education and promotion of consistent condom use remain the best prevention methods.

HIV/AIDS epidemics in many countries are concentrated in specific populations that are often marginalised and vulnerable to a broad range of health and psychosocial difficulties apart from, or in addition to, HIV/AIDS. Complex and interlinked factors influence their vulnerability.

i) Their socioeconomic circumstances (such as poverty, lack of education, displacement, separation from families, etc.) may hinder their ability to protect themselves, and may reduce their access to HIV prevention and care information, services and commodities.
ii) HIV prevalence among their social networks may be higher than in the general population.
iii) They may engage in specific high-risk behaviours such as sharing drug-injecting equipment or having unprotected sex with persons whose serostatus is unknown.

Such populations include injecting drug users, sex workers (and their clients), men who have sex with men, prisoners, marginalised young people, refugees and displaced persons, trafficked persons, socially excluded indigenous populations, and itinerant and mobile workers (such as seafarers, long-distance truck drivers and seasonal workers). Reaching these groups is vital for the success of an AIDS response. As many of these populations do not have access to mainstream HIV/AIDS services, outreach and peer network approaches must bring services to where they work, live and socialise. The most effective interventions and programmes are those that are tailored to the specific realities and needs of the people for whom they are intended.

In varying degrees, male-to-male HIV transmission is a factor in all HIV epidemics. It has been the predominant mode of transmission of HIV in most high-income countries. In the USA, male-to-male sex accounted for the largest proportion (42 per cent) of annual new infections in 2000, while, in Australia, it accounted for 54 per cent of infections in 2000. Significant HIV prevalence among men who have sex with men has been detected in countries around the world Where male-to-male sex is repressed legally or through strong social sanctions, men who have sex with men are at especially high risk of HIV infection, since they are harder to identify and reach with preventative services. Countering the discrimination and violence endured by men who have sex with men is therefore a vital part of an effective AIDS response.

Gay communities in high-income countries have been at the forefront of the response to HIV/AIDS, and have mounted very successful prevention efforts, although a resurgence of unsafe sex among men who have sex with men shows the need to constantly renew and reinforce such efforts. In much of Africa and Asia, however, prevention efforts among men who have sex with men have barely begun. In many middle and low-income countries, male-to-male sex and HIV transmission tend to be statistically hidden and officially denied. In much of Africa, for example, male-to-male sex is scarcely acknowledged, although self-identified gay groups have been in existence for several years in South Africa and Zimbabwe. Similar groups have recently been formed in Kenya and Senegal. The Bandhu Social

Welfare Society (in Dhaka, Bangladesh) and Sahodaran (in Chennai, India) are community based agencies providing both outreach and on site services to men who have sex with men. 'Safe spaces' in their central offices offer stigmatised and marginalised men an opportunity to socialise and to access a range of services. Bandhu Social Welfare Society has an innovative clinic service for sexually transmitted infection diagnosis and treatment and Sahodaran has contributed strongly to national advocacy. Similarly, recent years have seen a series of prevention projects established in Eastern Europe and Central Asia by gay organisations in collaboration with local authorities, with support from UNAIDS Cosponsors and the UNAIDS Secretariat. The projects are established in Minsk, Belarus; Bishkek, Kyrgyzstan; Karaganda and Almaty in Kazakhstan; and Tashkent in Uzbekistan. As in high-income countries, the solidarity of highly-placed or well-known individuals can be very helpful in fighting the stigma faced by this vulnerable population. In Haiti, for example, the country's First Lady recently gave public support to GRASADIS, which provides out-reach and peer education for men who have sex with men.

Injecting Drug Users

The illicit drug trade has, over the past 25 years, grown into a multi-billion-dollar industry that spans the planet. By the end of 1999, injecting drug use was being reported in 136 countries. In 114 of them, HIV cases resulting from injecting drug use had been reported. Drug trafficking is now a global phenomenon, touching some 170 countries and territories. It is estimated that up to 10 million people worldwide inject drugs. Asia is estimated to have the largest number of injecting-drug-related HIV cases. Injecting drug use is also a major factor in HIV epidemics in North America, Western Europe and in parts of Latin America, the Middle East and North Africa. In some Eastern European countries, especially in countries of the former Soviet Union, injecting drug use is driving major HIV/

AIDS epidemics among young people, and many outreach programmes report rising numbers of sexually active teenage drug users.

Injecting drug related HIV epidemics do not remain limited to injecting drug users. Most injecting drug users are young, male and sexually active. They are likely to acquire or transmit the HIV virus not only by sharing injecting equipment but also through sexual intercourse with regular or casual partners. Injecting drug use also overlaps profoundly with the sex trade, with users often buying sex, or selling sex to finance their drug dependencies. In 2000, in Hanoi, Viet Nam, 20 per cent of street based female sex workers reported recent drug injection, while 23 per cent of male injecting drug users bought sex; in Bangladesh, the corresponding figures were 14 per cent and 50–75 per cent respectively.

Preventing HIV Infection

Stopping the spread of HIV among injecting drug users requires a comprehensive approach, including drug dependency treatment and rehabilitation; HIV/AIDS education; access to clean needles/syringes and condoms; legal and social services; and voluntary HIV testing and counselling and psychosocial support. It also requires efforts to deter people (especially young people) from initiating injecting drug use. There is strong evidence to show that effective and humane drug treatment not only reduces drug abuse, but also diminishes HIV risk. A basic ethical principle is that drug control policies must reduce, not augment, the HIV risk faced by drug users, and HIV prevention activities must not inadvertently promote drug abuse. Small, isolated prevention efforts might slow the pace of the epidemic, but not for long, as Nepal's experience has shown. Needle exchange programmes there began as early as 1991; by 1995, some researchers were claiming that the interventions had averted a HIV epidemic among injecting drug users. But, by 1997, almost half the users tested in Kathmandu were infected with HIV.

The needle exchange programme was too limited and too localised to have a powerful, lasting impact. It had to be expanded. Needle and syringe programmes have also been expanded elsewhere, notably in some countries in Europe and in Australia. In 2000, in England and Wales, there were 420 syringe distribution programmes, distributing 27 million syringes, equivalent to 180 -540 syringes per injecting drug user per year.

Evidence from high and low income countries shows that effective prevention and care programmes can be mounted despite the marginalisation, social stigma and legally penalising environment that mark injecting drug users' lives. But the programmes tend to be most successful when laws and police practices facilitate outreach work and service provision to injecting drug users. For many years, Manipur in India was emblematic of a region in the grip of a rising injecting drug related HIV epidemic. By the late 1990s, there were already an estimated 40 000 injecting drug users in Manipur, as many as 60 per cent of whom were HIV-positive. To many observers, it seemed a 'lost cause'. But, after studies had revealed that most of the users shared injecting equipment because they feared arrest if caught with needles and syringes, the Society for HIV/AIDS and Lifelines Operations (SHALOM) took the bold step of setting up a needle and syringe exchange programme in Churachandpur township. Police were consulted and persuaded not to harass SHALOM workers or users found with injecting equipment. HIV incidence among users dropped from almost 77 per cent in 1997 to just under 59 per cent in 2001 still high, but a marked decrease. Persuaded by the effectiveness of the programme, the Manipur Minister of State for Health integrated the approach into the official State AIDS policy.

Bigger official obstacles were cleared in Ukraine, where, in 1998, the parliament added to a HIV/AIDS law the State's guarantee that it would work to facilitate the provision of needle-exchange services for injecting drug users. This hard won law reform also abolished the mandatory testing of users. Political and public opinion at first had been fearful that the changes would spur drug use and other social problems. But a strong information campaign and widespread public debate gradually convinced voters and legislators that the reforms were ultimately going to benefit all society.

In Brazil, a law was approved by Congress in 2002, authorising the Ministry of Health to establish national policies for specific HIV programmes targeting injecting drug users. A national survey among injecting drug users showed that consistent use of condoms in this population increased from 42 per cent in 1999 to 65 per cent in the year 2000. In the same period, syringe-and needle-sharing decreased from 70 per cent to 41 per cent. As a result, between 1996 and 2000, HIV prevalence among injecting drug users dropped in several cities. In Santos, Sao Paulo State, the drop was from 65 per cent to 42 per cent; in Salvador, from 49 per cent to 7 per cent; and in the city of Rio de Janeiro, from 25 per cent to 8 per cent.

Drug substitution programmes, along with a range of other health and referral services, have been successfully introduced in some places. An example is the Mexican non-governmental organisation, Companeros AC, which has run a programme since the mid 1990s, promoting detoxification and rehabilitation alongside specific HIV prevention efforts targeting injecting drug users. It helps injecting drug users make behavioural changes that are realistic for them and that are most likely to be sustained from outright cessation of drug use to adopting less harmful habits. Fieldwork is carried out in prisons as well as in the wider community. Information leaflets are distributed, along with packages containing condoms, bleach, and education leaflets. Rehabilitation services incorporate complementary treatments such as acupuncture and herbal medicine.

Education and support are provided to the families and partners of people who inject drugs. Removed from society, prisoners can be at special risk of HIV infection -mainly through injecting drug use, voluntary or forced sex, unsafe tattooing practices, and insufficient HIV prevention information, education and services. Many countries report at least some injecting drug use in prisons. Because needles are very difficult to obtain in these situations, sharing is particularly common and the potential for the spread of HIV significant. In Australia, about a quarter of prisoners inject drugs while incarcerated, according to a 2000 study. A study of 3200 imprisoned injecting drug users in seven European Union countries revealed that 45 per cent of the respondents had injected drugs in prison, and 7 per cent had started to inject while behind bars. Comparable statistics from low and middle income countries are less readily available. But some recent findings confirm anecdotal evidence that the risk of HIV infection through injecting drug use can be high. In Iran, for example, 10 prisons had reported HIV infection among injecting drug users by 2001, with one site reporting prevalence as high as 63 per cent. HIV prevalence of jailed injecting drug users in a prison in Bali, Indonesia, was reported at 53 per cent in 2000.

In an environment designed to administer legal punishments, it is not surprising that drug use by inmates is often met with further punishment. Yet this may backfire and even increase injecting drug use among prisoners. Research into mandatory drug screening in United Kingdom prisons found that inmates shifted from smoking marijuana (which is detectable in urine for several weeks) to injecting heroin (which disappears from urine after one or two days). Countries that, in the past, tried to counteract HIV transmission in prison with compulsory testing and isolation of HIV positive inmates are now revisiting those policies. Ukraine, for example, recently introduced a new policy based on extensive education, the introduction of voluntary counselling and testing, the integration of HIV-positive prisoners, and confidentiality regarding HIV status. Some prison systems are moving beyond offering information on HIV risks, towards safer injecting drug use by providing bleach to sterilise needles and syringes, making sterile needles available, and offering methadone maintenance treatment. Programmes addressing the specific needs of injecting drug users have also been supplemented with condom provision to reduce the sexual transmission of HIV.

Sex -consensual or forced among inmates is another source of risk of HIV infection, especially in countries where HIV spread is already substantial. In a survey conducted among 1100 male prisoners in Russia, only 10 –15 per cent of them reported having had no sexual contacts while incarcerated. A survey in Brazil found that 73 per cent of male prisoners had sex with other men in penal institutions. Forced sex was widespread. Consensual and forced sex with men is also the experience of many female inmates. Prisoners taking part in a study of New York State prisons and city jails, for example, reported frequent unprotected sex in prison, including between male prison officers and female inmates. Condom provision to prisoners is rare, except in Europe. By 2000, 16 high-income counters provided condoms in prisons. In Europe, the proportion of prison systems that had made condoms available rose from 53 per cent in 1989 to 81 per cent in 1997. In the most recent survey, condoms were available in all but four systems.

Sex Workers and their Clients

Sex work is clandestine and illegal in most societies, which makes it difficult to gauge the numbers involved in it. But it is a global phenomenon and a powerful social and economic factor in many countries. By the International Labour Organisation's estimates, the sex work industry accounted for more than 2 per cent of gross domestic product in four South-East Asian countries by the late 1990s. In countries where heterosexual intercourse is the main mode of HIV transmission, HIV epidemics tend to be concentrated initially among sex workers and their clients before becoming established in the wider population. A steep rise in HIV prevalence among sex workers is an alarm signal that HIV rates in the wider population are very likely to increase unless effective prevention efforts are introduced. Major shifts in HIV prevalence among antenatal clinic attendees lagged about half a decade behind, rising from 3 per cent in 1986, to 13. 8 per cent in 1999. Where sex work is widespread but clandestine, this often reflects entrenched gender inequaities. In such places, men's social, economic and political status eclipses that of women, double standards encourage multiple partners for men but not for women, and women's limited educational and livelihood opportunities compel many into some form of sex work. While economic necessity is often the driving motivation for many in sex work, it is not necessarily the only one. Research in the Philippine sex industry, for instance, has found that some sex workers operating out of bars and clubs had worked in formal employment, but opted instead for the slightly lower earnings and risks of the sex trade over the long hours working on assembly lines. Others are coerced into sex work through violence, debt bondage, or trafficking. The gap between knowing and doing It can be difficult or impossible for sex workers to insist on safe sex. Reluctant clients might react with violence or simply move on to someone willing to forego a condom.

A recent analysis of condom use by sex workers in Kolkata, India, has found that clients were willing to pay almost double the fee for sex without a condom. In parts of Indonesia, research shows that almost all sex workers know about HIV/AIDS and over three quarters know it can be avoided by using condoms. There is a significant mismatch between these women's knowledge and practice. Male clients were even less likely to always use condoms with sex workers, even though most knew that condoms could protect them from HIV and other sexually transmitted infections. The differences were consistent across the country.

Effective HIV prevention among sex workers addresses the social, economic and legal environments in which they live and work. Sex workers must be involved and empowered through the projects. Efforts must win the cooperation and support of control points in the sex industry, such as brothel owners, bar managers, pimps and the police. It is essential to tackle the prejudice that sex workers endure, and to weave other concerns into the programmes, such as care for their families and children.

The Sonagachi sex worker in Kolkata, India remains a benchmark example of this approach. About one-third of the 5000 sex workers operating there come from Bangladesh and Nepal. Most work out of brothels. Extensive surveys were done of sex workers, clients, boyfriends and sex workers 'children's needs. Sex workers themselves took part in the project's design and operation. Gradually, the scale and impact of the project grew, as women's groups, legal rights organisations and some government agencies backed the sex workers 'bids to reform the social system in which they worked. Sonagachi has been replicated in 30 red light districts reaching more than 31 000 sex workers in the state of West Bengal, and covering almost the entire state. The Sonagachi principle has also spread to Bangladesh, where both brothel and street based workers have been mobilised. Increasingly, in all these sites, sex workers 'communities have been involved in community development, non-formal education, community banking schemes, vocational training, and children's schooling.

When sex work is illegal, it is driven deeper underground, and prevention efforts become more difficult. Sex workers may be subject to police harassment, and carrying condoms can lead to arrest, fines or imprisonment. However, important victories have been won for the protection of sex workers' human rights. Sex workers involved in Bangladesh's SHAKTI project helped achieve an important court decision recognising sex work as a legal form of income-generation.

Uniformed Services

International and national uniformed services, including peacekeepers, peace observers, national defence and civil defence forces, generally rank among the population groups most affected by sexually transmitted infections, including

HIV/AIDS. In peacetime, sexually transmitted infection rates among armed forces are generally two-to-five times higher than in the general populace. This difference can be much greater in times of conflict, with infection rates increasing as much as 50 times.

Several aspects of the military environment put its armed forces personnel at risk, including the fact that most soldiers are in the age group at greatest risk of HIV infection as well as the ethos of risk-taking that characterises the military. Yet, one of the most important factors that increase the risk of infection is the practice of posting personnel away from their own communities and families. Not only does this free soldiers from the discipline they might be subject to in their own communities, but it also removes them from their spouses or regular sexual partners. The resulting loneliness, stress and sexual tension increase risk-taking. A study of Dutch soldiers on a five-month peacekeep-vices, and rates of 50 -60 per cent in countries where HIV/AIDS has been present for more than a decade.

According to a US National Intelligence Council document, the military cost of AIDS is likely to be highest among the more modernised armed forces in sub-Saharan Africa, and especially in their officer ranks. As more officers and key personnel fall ill, the combat readiness and capability of such military forces are expected to deteriorate. HIV/AIDS also jeopardises the families and communities of military personnel. In many countries, a large number of young males either volunteer for, or are conscripted into, military services. When defence and civil defence forces are demobilised, there is a risk of broadening the spread of HIV.

Military and other uniformed services need to address HIV/AIDS within their ranks and among those they have a mandate to protect. Changing the perception and behaviour of soldiers, police officers, border and customs officials can produce significant benefits for the general population. This is especially true in countries affected by war or civil unrest. Uniformed services also represent a unique opportunity for providing HIV prevention and education to a large 'captive' and influential audience particularly the new young recruits, who represent an important peer group both within the uniformed services and their own wider communities.

An important first step in defending against AIDS is to create a non-stigmatising and nondiscriminatory environment. This begins with full confidentiality for HIV testing something not every country supports. The Panel stressed that voluntary counselling and testing should be provided to peacekeeping personnel and should be offered as part of a comprehensive range of integrated HIV prevention and care services.

New Prevention Technologies

Potential technologies currently being pursued also hold the promise of radically changing the landscape of HIV/AIDS prevention. Most prominent are microbicides and vaccines against HIV. As a form of 'chemical condom' that can be self-administered, microbicides could increase the options for women and men who find it difficult or impossible to persuade their partners to use a condom.

Acceptability studies in South Africa, Uganda and Zimbabwe suggest that women who seldom or never use condoms could reduce their overall risk of infection if an effective microbicide were available to them at low cost. Applied inside the vagina or rectum, a micro-bicide is intended to prevent infection with HIV and, possibly, other bacterial and viral sexually transmitted infections. It can be produced as a gel, cream, suppository, sponge or in other forms, and may also have contraceptive properties. The ideal product would be odourless and colourless, and therefore undetectable to partners who refuse other forms of protection.

After the disappointment of the Phase III trial of nonoxynol-9 gel, an estimated 56 new products are in various stages of development, from pre-clinical stages to Phase III effectiveness trials. While no major pharmaceutical company has thus far invested in the development of a microbicide, research into this preventive option has recently been spurred by several grants from the Bill and Melinda Gates Foundation. The International Working Group on Microbicides, which includes public agencies from around the world among its members, continues to promote and facilitate the development of microbicides.

Vaccines: Research to find a vaccine against HIV has been making steady progress in the past 10 years. Unfortunately, 'steady' is not fast enough for all the people who could benefit from it. Even if current attempts to speed up the research process and programmes for the introduction of vaccines are successful, there is little chance that vaccination against HIV will be available on a large scale before the end of the decade.

An estimated US$400 -500 million is currently spent on HIV vaccine research annually, with most of this going into basic research. Institutions involved in the global HIV vaccine effort include the US National Institutes of Health, the International AIDS Vaccine Initiative (IAVI), the US Centers for Disease Control and Prevention, the French Agence Nationale de Recherches sur le SIDA (ANRS), the European Community (through the EUROVAC programme), and several biotechnology and pharmaceutical companies. National AIDS vaccine research programmes are ongoing in Australia, Canada, Japan, Sweden, the United Kingdom and the United States of America. Low and middle income countries are also actively involved in vaccine development and trials. WHO and UNAIDS have been actively supporting these national AIDS vaccine programmes.

Despite all this activity, the peculiarities of the HIV virus make finding a vaccine difficult and expensive. HIV differs from most other infectious diseases in that the virus directly attacks white blood cells that are central to directing the body's immune responses, leaving them incapable of controlling infection or preventing disease. 'Classical' vaccines, based on an entire microorganism (viruses or bacteria) that has been killed or rendered harmless, may not be safe enough to use against HIV as they could lead to HIV infection. Experimental HIV vaccines are therefore primarily based on parts of the virus, which makes the development of a vaccine even more challenging.

The multiple variants of HIV pose a further complication. Ten subtypes of the HIV-1 virus have been identified, and are distributed in different parts of the world. Researchers do not yet know whether a broadly protective vaccine will be possible or if a separate vaccine will be needed for each subtype. The most prevalent HIV subtypes are A and C, present in different regions in Africa, but the majority of the vaccines currently in trials are modelled on the genetic profile of subtype B -the one predominant in high-income countries.

Finally, HIV vaccine research remains a 'high-risk/low-return investment' for private sector industry. This is only partly because the greatest need for the vaccine is among low-income countries. An even greater obstacle at least currently is the inadequate scientific understanding of the mechanisms by which the virus evades the body's natural immune responses. Consequently, it is not known exactly what immune responses are necessary to prevent or control HIV infection.

Developing a HIV vaccine is an arduous process. Experimental vaccines are first tested on animals, and the best vaccine candidates are then selected for possible testing on humans. Testing is then carried out on healthy volunteers in three phases.

Phase I trials are done on 20–40 volunteers to confirm the vaccine's safety and whether it triggers useful HIV-specific immune responses.

Phase II tests involve hundreds of volunteers to further check safety and assess the potency of immune responses.

Phase III tests can last up to four years and involve field trials with thousands of volunteers, some of whom receive the vaccine while others form a control group. Extremely complicated from the logistical, scientific and ethical points of view, these trials assess whether the candidate vaccine protects against HIV infection or the onset of AIDS.

AIDS AND HUMAN RIGHTS

HIV/AIDS has burrowed deeper into the social and economic fault lines of communities and societies, and it is widening those fissures further. Around the world, those most affected by HIV/AIDS are people and communities who have unequal access to fundamental social and economic rights. The denial of basic rights limits people's options to defend their autonomy, develop viable livelihoods and protect themselves, leaving them more vulnerable to both HIV infection and the impact of the epidemic on their lives. It is therefore necessary to assess the epidemic in the context of human rights. Viewing the epidemic in this way also brings into sharper relief some of the prerequisites for an effective response: integrating principles, norms and standards as established in existing international human rights instruments, and using national and international rights institutions to realise these rights.

Human rights that relate critically to reducing vulnerability to HIV/AIDS and mitigating the impact of the epidemic are found in existing human rights instruments, such as the Universal Declaration on Human Rights, the Covenant on Economic, Social and Cultural Rights the Covenant on Civil and Political Rights, the Convention on the Elimination of all Forms of Discrimination against Women, and the Convention on the Rights of the Child.

Principles of nondiscrimination, equality and participation are central to an effective HIV/AIDS strategy that integrates human rights. More specifically, the most relevant human rights principles for protecting the dignity of people infected and affected by HIV/AIDS, as well as preventing the spread of infection, include: nondiscrimination; the right to health; the right to equality between men and women; the rights of children; the right to privacy; the right to education and information; the right to work; the right to marry and found a family; the right to social security, assistance and welfare; the right to liberty; and the right to freedom of movement.

In the context of HIV/AIDS, governments have the obligation to respect, protect and fulfil human rights. A framework of accountability exists through the series of international instruments established over the past 50 years. Indeed, the past two years have seen wider recognition of HIV/AIDS-related interpretations of human rights frameworks:

i) *General comment 14 on the right to health,* adopted by the Committee on Economic, Social and Cultural Rights, situates several key features of the right to health within the context of HIV/AIDS. These include the availability and acceptability of, and access to, functioning public health-care facilities, goods and services, and programmes.
ii) *The UN Commission on Human Rights Resolution 2001/33 on 'Access to medication in the context of pandemics such as HIV/AIDS'* recognises that access to medication in the context of epidemics such as HIV/AIDS is fundamental to achieving the full realisation of the right to the highest attainable standard of physical and mental health; the resolution calls upon States to pursue policies that pro- mote the availability of HIV/AIDS-related medications in sufficient quantities and in ways that make them accessible to all.

The international human rights framework provides a solid basis for individuals and organisations to drive home their demands for change and action, to claim and exercise their rights, to resist exclusion and marginalisation, and to struggle for social justice.

Unequal access to life-saving HIV treatments is a glaring human rights issue. It also affects the degree of stigma that persists, since HIV- related stigma and discrimination are largely due to the fact that HIV/AIDS is seen as incurable. Increasing access to medications therefore not only helps to realise the right to health and overcome inequities due to poverty it also changes attitudes. Deploying rights principles, norms and standards, activists have won ground-breaking victories on this front. In Costa Rica, local non-governmental organisations helped a HIV-positive college student file a petition with the Supreme Court demanding combination therapy, which he could not afford. The court ruled in his favour triggering a dozen similar petitions. Within weeks, the national social security system was ordered to develop a plan for the provision of antiretroviral treatment to all citizens living with HIV/AIDS.

In Venezuela, Accion Ciudadana Contra el SIDA, together with health professionals, lawyers and AIDS activists, filed a suit in 1997 on behalf of a group of people living with HIV/ AIDS who were covered by the Social Security Protecting people at risk and those who are vulnerable System. The lawsuit alleged that the claimants were not receiving proper medical attention, as guaranteed by the National Constitution, the American Convention on Human Rights, and other conventions signed and ratified by Venezuela. The court upheld the lawsuit and ordered the Social Security System to provide free treatment to the plaintiffs. Countries in other regions are beginning to follow these examples as they move to realise the rights of people living with HIV/AIDS.

Groups affected by societal discrimination include women and children and, in many places, racial and ethnic groups, migrants and refugees. Other groups suffer discrimination because the activities they engage in are subject to criminal sanctions or social disapproval.

Such people include those with different sexual orientations, as well as sex workers, drug users and prisoners. For example, globally, a significant share of HIV infection occurs in male-to-male sex. Yet, dozens of countries still maintain laws that explicitly prohibit or regulate same-sex sexual relations. The effect is often that of stripping men who have sex with men of vital rights (including the right to access information and services that can protect them from the virus), leaving them highly vulnerable.

Around the world, women's enhanced physiological risk of HIV infection is compounded by economic deprivation, lack of employment opportunities, poor access to education, training and information, and sociocultural norms and practices. In sub-Saharan Africa, for example, prevalence among teenage girls in some countries is five times higher than that for teenage boys. Most of these infections occur as a result of unprotected heterosexual intercourse. Women's low economic and social status limits their power to negotiate the use of a condom, discuss fidelity with their partners, or leave risky relationships. Such disempowerment increases their vulnerability to HIV; the socioeconomic and sexual discrimination thus experienced by women can ultimately become life-threatening.

Research underscores these realities. In a study in Viet Nam, only 35% of women felt able to refuse their husbands sex, while a UNIFEM study on the impact of HIV/AIDS on communities in Zimbabwe revealed that, even if women were educated about HIV/AIDS, their economic dependence on men left them feeling 'helpless' to negotiate safe sex. Sexual coercion and violence in all its forms, inside and outside marriage, in peacetime and in conflict, increase the threat of HIV infection for women and girls. In population-based studies worldwide, 10-50% of women report physical assault by an intimate partner, and between one-third and one-half of physically abused women also report sexual coercion.

Indigenous women, refugees and displaced women, women of certain religious groups, women in migration and trafficked women are also among those most vulnerable, with the attendant HIV/AIDS risks. The impact of war on women and young girls can be particularly severe, with the relatively recent experiences of Bosnia, Croatia and Rwanda revealing again how rape and other forms of sexual abuse are frequently used as weapons of war.

Policies that reduce people's vulnerability and make it easier for them to choose safer behaviour are vital for an effective AIDS response. Income-generation schemes, improving women's employment opportunities and micro-finance schemes are among the potential options for boosting women's economic independence. Among many such initiatives are those of ILO, which is strengthening microfinance and entrepreneurial skills among women in Malawi, Mozambique, the United Republic of Tanzania and Zimbabwe.

Evidence in relation to condom negotiation, voluntary counselling and testing, and the uptake of interventions to prevent HIV transmission from mother to child points in the same direction: women's empowerment and safety depend also on changes in the attitudes and deeds of men and boys. The 2000 -2001 World AIDS Campaign was aimed at involving men more fully in the fight against AIDS.

Fighting AIDS Discrimination

The protection of human rights is critical to reducing the impact of the epidemic on people living with HIV/AIDS. Historically, AIDS discrimination was first witnessed in the victimisation of seropositive individuals and in the intolerance and social ostracism inflicted on them. While these abuses regrettably still occur in all countries, responses based both on humanitarian and pragmatic considerations have been developed, and the list of successful HIV/AIDS-related human rights activism efforts has grown impressively.

In Mumbai, India, for example, the Lawyers Collective has successfully defended workers who lost their jobs on account of their HIV status. The Collective also raises public awareness about HIV/AIDS through public rallies, and mobilises public opinion against stigma and discrimination. One of its significant achievements has been the upholding of a clause that allows people with HIV/AIDS to file their cases under a pseudonym. In New Delhi, meanwhile, the Population Council is helping set up HIV-Patient-Friendly Hospitals. The goal is to make hospitals more attuned to the needs of people with HIV/AIDS.

And in South Africa, the Centre for the Study of AIDS at the University of Pretoria is working to foster a climate for a sustained and effective response to HIV/AIDS on the campus and in society in general. By placing the epidemic in a human rights context, and by challenging stigma, discrimination, racism and prejudices, the University hopes to enable staff and students to freely disclose their HIV status, should they wish to do so. Students receive training in all aspects of HIV/AIDS and are actively supported in their efforts to counter HIV/AIDS-related stigma and discrimination in their communities.

National human rights institutions in Ghana, India and South Africa have launched activities that promote and protect HIV/AIDS-related human rights in their countries. Legislators are also advancing HIV/AIDS- related human rights. The United Kingdom Westminster All-Party Parliamentary Group on HIV/AIDS, for example, held public hearings in 2001 to identify legal and policy reforms to be introduced in the next five years. At a regional level, the Southern African Development Community (SADC) Parliamentary Forum has set up a Standing Committee on HIV/AIDS, which is developing strategic work plans to address HIV/AIDS-related issues.

Beyond Stigma and Discrimination

Widespread HIV/AIDS-related stigma and discrimination persist, despite the fact that they increase people's vulnerability and, by isolating people and depriving them of care and support, worsen the impact of infection. Indeed, they impede every step in an effective response, from prevention, to treatment, care and support, and even extend into the next generation, placing an emotional burden on children who may also be trying to cope with the death of their parents, due to AIDS.

But stigma and discrimination do not arise in a vacuum. They emerge from, and reinforce, other stereotypes, prejudices and social inequalities, including those relating to gendernationality, ethnicity and sexuality, as well as activities that are criminalised (such as sex work, drug use or male-male sex). Stigma, discrimination and human rights violations form a vicious circle, legitimising and spurring each other. With its focus on stigma and discrimination, the 2002 -2003 World AIDS Campaign aims to spur action against stigma and discrimination, as part of worldwide efforts that include:

i) encouraging leaders at all levels, and in all walks of life, to visibly challenge HIV- related discrimination, spearhead public action and act against the many other forms of discrimination that people face in relation to HIV/AIDS;
ii) actively involving people living wit h HIV/AIDS in the response to the epidemic; monitoring violations of human rights,
iii) and ensuring that people are able to challenge discrimination and receive redress through national administrative, judicial and human rights institutions designed to safeguard rights;
iv) creating an enabling legal environment for fighting discrimination; and ensuring that prevention and treatment, care and support services are accessible to all.

An effective, long-term response to the epidemic hinges on the recognition and protection of people's rights. Individuals and communities who are able to realise their rights to information, education, health and health care, and who are protected against discrimination and violence, are less vulnerable to the epidemic.

In 2000-2001, UNAIDS, in collaboration with the International Council of AIDS Service Organisations and its regional structures, concentrated on strengthening civil society capacity to realise and protect HIV/AIDS- related human rights. Working with the Asia Pacific Council of AIDS Service Organisations, UNAIDS developed a training module on human rights and HIV/AIDS for that region, and conducted training in Cambodia. The Latin American Council of AIDS Service Organisations, meanwhile, held a regional workshop to identify the human rights implications of National AIDS strategic plans in the region, and devised strategies to integrate human rights activities into those plans. And the African Council of AIDS Service Organisations is supporting community-based activities aimed at integrating human rights into prevention and care efforts in Burkina Faso and the United Republic of Tanzania.

Some of the most successful responses to the epidemic have occurred when people, ranging from gay communities in high-income countries, starting in the 1980s, to urban and rural communities in Uganda, and sex workers in Bangladesh and India, have seized the right to speak out, mobilise resources and organise.

In Bangladesh, sex workers have joined in a collective called Durjoy, which combats the trafficking of girls and young women in the sex industry. Along with nongovernmental organisations, Durjoy in 2001 won a court judgement that legally recognised the rights of sex workers to practise their trade and sup- port their families. In Kolkata, India, mean-while, sex workers have gone a step further and now build skills among local police to combat violence against them. In addition, they have created a board that brings together sex workers, local sex industry operators and government labour and health authorities to tackle violence in the industry.

The activism of civil society around rights issues remains one of the sterling features of effective responses everywhere, especially when it involves people living with and affected by HIV/AIDS, and young people. In a range of African and Asian countries, the UNAIDS Secretariat is supporting training for national partners on HIV/AIDS-related human rights for community AIDS organisations, human rights non-governmental organisations, political leaders, National AIDS Programme managers, people living with HIV/AIDS, and legislators.

REFERENCES

UNAIDS, Report on the Global HIV/AIDS Epidemic, 2002.

WHO, World Health Report, 2001.

Bibliography

A Situational Assessment of HIV/AIDS in the Maldives for the Year 2000, UN Theme Group on HIV/AIDS, 2000.

Bhutan Ministry of Social Services, Medium Term Plan and Control of AIDS in Bhutan, 1990-1993, WHO Report, 1993.

Cockerell, C. J., Cutaneous and historic signs of HIV infection other than Kaposi's sarcoma. In G. P. Wormser (ed.), *AIDS and other manifestations of HIV infection,* New York: Raven Press, 1992.

Fernando N., *Migrant Women Workers,* Sri Lanka.

Finley, J. L., Joshi, V. V., & Neil, J. S. A., General pathology of HIV infection. In G. P. Wormser (ed.)*AIDS and other manifestations of HIV infection.* New York: Raven Press, 1992.

Fischl, M. A., Treatment of HIV infection, In M. A. Sande & P. A. Volberding (eds.), *The medical management of AIDS.* Philadelphia: Saunders, 1992.

Gordon, G., and T. Klouda, *Preventing a Crisis: AIDS and Family Planning Work:* London: International Planned Parenthood Federation, 1989.

Government of Bangladesh, *Strategic Plan of the Natioinal AIDS Programmes of Bangladesh, 1997-2002,* July 2000.

Government of Nepal, Strategic Plan for HIV and AIDS in Nepal 1997-2001, Final Draft, July, 2002.

HIV/AIDS in Asia and the Pacific Region, 2001, WHO Report, 2001.

HIV/AIDS Surveillance Database, US Census Beuro, 2001.

Human Development Repot, 2001.

Kundu B. Mitra A., Kar J., Ghosh P., July-September 2000, *AIDS: An Indian Experience,* Srishti, A Bhoruka Public Welfare Trust Publication, Calcutta, India.

Lama M.P., Managing Refugees in South Asia, 2000. Bangladesh: Refugee and Migratory Movements Research Unit.

Ministry of Health, Republic of Maldives, Health Master Plan 1996-2005.

NACO, HIV /AIDS India Scenario, 2001.

_______________ , Comabting HIV/AIDS in India, 2000-2001.

NCASC, Situational Analysis of HIV/AIDS in Nepal, NCASC, Ministry of Health, Kathmandu, December, 2000.

Nishimizu, Mieko, "Sri Lanka, AIDS and Development", *The Daily Mirror*, Sri Lanka, October 29, 2002.

Rao A., April 1997, *Report of Workshop on Indo-Nepal Cross Border Intervention Strategy on HIV/AIDS,* Bhoruka Public Welfare Trust, Calcutta, India.

Rasheeda A., Maldives Country Paper for 11th Meeting of National AIDS Programme Managers, Jakarta, 1995.

Report of the UN Secretary General, August 1999, *Violence Against Women Migrant Workers,* New York

Report on *Regional Retreat on Migration Strategy and Vulnerability to HIV/AIDS,* UNDP, January 2001, Sri Lanka: Institute for Participatory Interaction in Development (IPID).

Report on South Asian Consultation on Economic Reforms and Migration with Special Focus on Women Workers, Centre for Education and Communication, February 2001, New Delhi, India.

Sentinel Surveillance Data Resources, Department of Health, Myanmar, March, 1988.

Sierra Health Foundation, *Challenge for the future: Coordinating HIV/AIDS care and services in the next decade.* Rancho Cordova, 1991.

South Asia HIV/AIDS Overview, The World Bank Reprot, 2002.

Sri Lanka, National STD/AIDS Control Sentinel Surveillance Reports, 1994, 1995, 1996, National AIDS Prevention and Control Programme, Ministry of Health, Sri Lanka.

UNAIDS Report on the Global HIV/AIDS Epidemic, 2002.

WHO, World Health Report, 2001.

WHO's Report on HIV/AIDS in Asia and the Pacific region, 2001.

Index